SPRING Forward

Many female athletes struggle with body confidence and change their nutrition in unhealthy ways, only to the detriment of both their performance and their health. *SPRING Forward: Balanced Eating, Exercise, and Body Image in Sport for Female Athletes* provides performance nutrition and body image flexibility guidance for adolescent and adult female athletes. This book details the problems and the consequences, and provides extensive education on healthier, higher-quality performance.

Nutritional details include specific nutritional needs for female athletes related to hormones and nutrition for peak performance, as well as fad diets. Body image education includes societal pressure, unrealistic ideals, handling mental aspects of body image, psychological obstacles, and dealing with more severe problems. Healthy performance is addressed along with sleep, camaraderie, and how to manage the ups and downs of being a female athlete.

Several instructional manuals that can be easily used for teams at any level, from secondary school to elite athletes, are included in the book. Secondary school athletes who used the program showed significant improvement in body image flexibility and gave the program rave reviews, stating that not only were they stronger athletes, but their teams also felt the education was a bonding experience.

Kathryn Vidlock is an Associate Professor at Rocky Vista University College of Osteopathic Medicine. She is fellowship trained in primary care sports medicine. She has been the team physician for the University of Iowa and many other teams as well as serving as medical director for numerous running and triathlon events. Dr. Vidlock has worked with athletes from the recreational level to elites–Olympic qualifiers and professional levels. She was an All-American Collegiate swimmer and understands the mind-set of athletes. She has worked with athletes and fueling for performance for over 20 years.

Catherine Liggett is a medical student at the University of Colorado. She and Dr. Vidlock are the cofounders of the research behind the principles in the SPRING Forward program. She was an Academic All-Big 12 first-team cross-country and track athlete at the University of Kansas and had numerous outstanding performances at Big 12 championships. Prior to starting medical school, she worked at a sports medicine office where she was involved in care of athletes performing at all levels of competition from recreational to professional. Following completion of medical school, she hopes to pursue a career where she can continue to work with athletes and promote education on balanced eating and exercise within sport.

Andrew Dole is a Registered Dietitian currently working with the New Zealand Olympic rugby teams, as well as numerous elite endurance athletes on an individual level. As a certified executive chef, sports dietician, and sports scientist, he combines his skills into performance-driven plans. He is currently working on his PhD studying nutrition with female ultra-endurance runners at the University of Waikato, New Zealand.

SPRING Forward

Balanced Eating, Exercise, and Body Image in Sport for Female Athletes

Kathryn Vidlock
Catherine Liggett
Andrew Dole

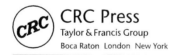

CRC Press
Taylor & Francis Group
Boca Raton London New York

CRC Press is an imprint of the
Taylor & Francis Group, an **informa** business

First edition published 2023
by CRC Press
6000 Broken Sound Parkway NW, Suite 300, Boca Raton, FL 33487-2742

and by CRC Press
4 Park Square, Milton Park, Abingdon, Oxon, OX14 4RN

CRC Press is an imprint of Taylor & Francis Group, LLC

© 2023 Taylor & Francis Group, LLC

ISBN: 978-1-032-38568-6 (hbk)
ISBN: 978-1-032-38564-8 (pbk)
ISBN: 978-1-003-34565-7 (ebk)

DOI: 10.1201/b23228

Typeset in Times
by SPi Technologies India Pvt Ltd (Straive)

Contents

Introduction

Kathryn Vidlock

Most athetes know that disordered eating and decreased body image are present in almost every sport. Many times it is hidden; nobody wants to talk about it. Athletes constantly strive to fit into a body-type ideal that isn't realistic. Education is the way to stop this in its tracks.

The authors are athletes who have all either experienced some of the issues, or know athletes that have dealt with it. We recognize that these issues are universal, affecting cisgendered, transgendered, and nonbinary female athletes of all races, ethnicities, socioeconomic status, religious/spiritual beliefs, backgrounds, and sexual preferences. We are passionate about making sure that all current and future female athletes are more knowledgeable and able to make healthy mental and physical decisions.

This book stems from that passion. In this book, we provide a background of the issue, explain the risks, discuss body image, disprove body image myths, provide nutrition and well-being information, and above all, empower female athletes to be the best person they can be. In addition, we have a template of this information in session form to share with teams or small groups of athletes. This project started with high school athletes, but there was such a great response from collegiate athletes and adult recreational athletes that we have added a session manual for athletes beyond the high school level. No matter your level of sport, recreational to elite, or your age, we hope you find this information helpful.

We asked athletes to share their stories and there were a plethora of responses. We will share some throughout the book. The names have been changed for anonymity.

AN ATHLETE'S STORY: Hallie

I have always loved sports. Growing up, I was involved in swimming, soccer, tennis, and overly competitive neighborhood games. In middle school, I became serious about soccer and considered it my main sport until sophomore year of high school when I transitioned to competitive year-round swimming. Because I had invested significant time and energy into soccer for several years, it was difficult to end that chapter. Although I was no longer enjoying practice and games as I once had, I hung on for a long time because I didn't want to be a quitter or let anyone down (people pleaser to the core). It is important to note that throughout my sports career prior to competitive swimming, I did not exhibit any disordered eating behaviors. With a blank slate (or pristine pool) ahead of me, I went "all in". During the last two years of high school, I was dedicated to becoming the strongest, fastest swimmer I could be. I practiced before and after school multiple days a week and started lifting weights. I also changed how I was eating, with top performance in mind. Little did I know it was the beginning of a rigid and harmful relationship with food and fueling that would persist and worsen for years to come. At first, I limited ingredients that I termed "unhealthy" or "bad"—mostly fat and sugar. I was unaware of how my drive to be "healthy" and to perform well could have significant negative consequences.

Period! Yes, there were ramifications for that pesky, inconvenient monthly cycle. With pain, cramps, and bloating it isn't always a female's best friend, especially female athletes. So, when mine became irregular, and eventually disappeared altogether I wasn't too concerned—huge mistake! A female's cycle is a critical indicator of adequate fueling, health and well-being. Even though it might have been "easier" to not have a period while training and competing, I now know I was not giving my body adequate energy to perform, which is detrimental to performance and overall health.

In August 2014, after completing a great season (meeting goals and achieving several personal bests), I said goodbye to high school and my menstrual cycle.

My fastest times took place in the first semester of freshman year. After that, I did not see time improvements in any of my events throughout the remaining three and a half years of competing. That was not because I didn't train hard. In fact, I scheduled extra sessions in the weight room with our trainer. I stayed after practice because "more is better". Right? WRONG! Because I was not fueling my body appropriately for the amount of activity, my performance severely declined. Was I having fun? No. I was constantly freezing in practice and in races because my body had no reserves to keep warm. I lost weight (including muscle) and was easily agitated and irritable. Why did I keep going? Because I wanted control. I didn't know how to effectively cope with the stress and expectations I placed on myself to be perfect—to be the best athlete, student, friend, sister, daughter, etc. So, I continued to use food as my source of "control". Looking back, it is ironic to see how much food was controlling me. My rigid habits persisted, and my list of "unhealthy" and "bad" foods expanded. By the end of college, I was basically eating as "clean" as possible. These behaviors were internal choices I made but were reinforced by comments from teammates at the dining hall—"You are SO healthy, I don't know how you do it, I wish I had your willpower".

Searching for some sense of identity as my performance declined, I then incorporated other's view of me as "the healthy one". It saddens me to think about how much time and energy I spent during college thinking about food to comply with all the rules I had created. This time and energy could have been spent being more present with friends and teammates and enjoying being a college student and athlete. In my experience, restricting/controlling food did not lead to extraordinary performance and happiness. In fact, it did the opposite.

My intention is not to scare or worry you. Rather, I hope my experience with disordered eating inspires you to give YOUR body what it needs to function, perform, and thrive! I want to see you achieve your goals and have fun along the way!

You are not alone. It is easy to be overwhelmed and influenced by the constant new diet trends, workout crazes, and health information we are exposed to constantly. I truly want you to be your healthiest, strongest, happiest self— full of confidence, power, and determination. I want you to be excited about who you are and love your unique self. I want this for me too, so let's do this together. Let's overcome the desire to fit a mold of what we are "supposed to eat" or "supposed to look like". Let's release our need to be perfect. Let's find healthy ways to manage stress. Let's accept our worthiness as human beings, not based on how we look or what we accomplish. Let's embrace our individuality. Let's be there for one another and lift each other up as we break free from rules, restrictions, and expectations.

With love, support, and encouragement,
Hallie

1 Background

Kathryn Vidlock
Rocky Vista University, Parker, CO, USA

Catherine Liggett
University of Colorado School of Medicine, Aurora, CO, USA

Nicole Oberlag
Claremont College, Claremont, CA, USA

Biana Gershman
HealthONE Family Medicine Residency, Aurora, CO, USA

CONTENTS

WORDS TO KNOW

FEMALE ATHLETE TRIAD   Older term consisting of disordered eating and lower energy availability, irregular menstrual cycles and hormonal imbalances, and decreased bone density and osteoporosis.

RELATIVE ENERGY DEFICIENCY IN SPORT (RED-S)   A syndrome caused by energy deficiency, potentially impacting metabolism, hormones, menstrual function, bone health, immunity, protein synthesis, and heart function.

HISTORY

Christy Henrich seemed to have an extremely successful gymnastics career. She was an All-Around silver medal winner in the US National Championships and placed fourth in the World Championships. But that same year, one of the judges at an international event told her she was fat and needed to lose weight. That comment spurred an eating disorder. By age 22, she was down to 47 pounds and passed away after multiple organs failed to function.[1] Christy's death received media attention and helped initiate education aimed to prevent eating disorders. Although that death happened in 1994, issues with female athletes dealing with unhealthy body image and eating disorders continue, and there are still examples of famous athletes who have had these struggles today.

Mary Cain was a national sensation in the world of running, breaking multiple records and being the youngest American athlete to qualify for World Championships. In 2013, she joined the most elite track team at the time, Nike's Oregon Project. From that point on Cain's performance and mental health began to deteriorate, as she was constantly told by coaches that she needed to lose weight. She was told that to be faster she needed to be thinner, and this took a toll on her physical and mental performance. Cain lost her period for three years and broke five bones, as well as became suicidal and began cutting. In 2019, Cain spoke out against Nike and her former coach Alberto Salazar, attempting to cause change in a system that halted her athletic career and put her own health at risk. Cain's statement and charges have inspired many other athletes to come forward with their own struggles, helping to grow the fight against this toxic culture in female sports.[2]

One of the athletes inspired by Cain is Lauren Fleshman. Fleshman is an incredibly accomplished athlete. She ran collegiately at Stanford, where she won five national titles and was a 15-time All-American. Luckily, Fleshman had a coach that supported positive body image and healthy eating habits. But that doesn't negate the fact that Fleshman was surrounded by a culture of eating disorders for most of her running career. She recalled at the 1998 National Foot Locker Cross Country Championships that many of the other girls ate a pre-race meal of only a salad with dressing on the side. When Fleshman transitioned to a pro runner, she restricted her diet in an attempt to fit the archetype female runner (very thin and lean). She ended up underfueling, losing her period, injuring herself, and hurting the beginning of her professional career. Fleshman is now a strong advocate of changing this harmful culture in female sports. She argues that the current sports system is built for men's bodies rather than the development of women's bodies. Fleshman also calls out the role coaches play in perpetuating this negative environment and the need for change.[3]

Amy Yoder Begley was another member of Nike's Oregon Project and a runner who was harmed by the pressure to lose weight in order to succeed. Yoder Begley was an Indiana state champion in cross county and at 3200 meters in high school track and later ran at the University of Arkansas, where she won two NCAA championships and was a 15-time All-American. In 2004 she won the 10 km road racing national championships, then joined Nike's Oregon Project in 2007. However, Yoder Begley was constantly criticized for her weight, and if she had a bad workout her coaches would blame it on her looking flabby. This continued throughout her training, with Yoder Begley starving herself, being pitted against teammates, and experiencing deteriorating mental health. In 2011, Yoder Begley was kicked off the Nike team after multiple injuries and Salazar telling her she had "the biggest butt on the start line". Shortly after, Yoder Begley lost funding and ended her professional career.[3]

Kara Goucher is a professional endurance runner who has also come forward with her struggles with disordered eating. Goucher is a three-time NCAA Champion from the University of Colorado and an Olympic medal winner. In an interview with FloTrack, Goucher revealed that she had problems with eating in college. She explained how she was only eating a granola bar and dinner per day; the breaking point was when she refused to eat a Dorito on a date with her now husband Adam Goucher, who is also a professional runner.[4] Goucher was lucky enough to have the support of Adam and her family to overcome these problems and went on to have a successful career. Later Goucher was part of Nike's Oregon Project. In 2011, she first came forward with concerns about doping within Nike's Oregon Project after Salazar gave her unprescribed Cytomel, a drug that treats underactive thyroid, to lose weight after a pregnancy. Goucher is now considered a whistleblower after an investigation was launched on the project in 2015.[5] In January 2020, Goucher published *#REDS (Relative Energy Deficiency in Sport): time for a revolution in sports culture and systems to improve athlete health and performance* along with Cain and Fleshman to bring more attention to this issue.[6]

These struggles and patterns are not limited to the sport of running and have been experienced by many famous athletes. Gracie Gold was a teenage ice skating sensation. In 2014, Gold won a national title, a bronze medal in a team event and a fourth-place finish in women's singles at the Olympics. She was projected to win the gold medal in the 2018 Olympics. However, Gold faced many setbacks as she struggled with mental health and eating disorders. She had a coach tell her that her weight was a large number, which pushed Gold to limit her caloric intake. Due to her competitive nature, she committed to having only a few hundred calories a day and soon fell into a binge-purge eating cycle. Gold struggled with weight gain and developed depression and suicidal thoughts. She finally reached out for help and decided to take a break from the sport.[7]

In 2014, Yulia Lipnitskaya became one of the youngest Olympic skating gold medalists when she won the team title with Russia at the age of 15. She was a national sensation and a very decorated skater. However, Lipnitskaya retired shortly after the Olympics due to anorexia. She entered a clinic to receive help and decided to retire from the sport. Due to her struggles with disordered eating and body image, and this culture within her sport, Lipnitskaya stepped away, choosing to put her personal health first.[8]

Amanda Beard is a seven-time Olympic gold medalist in swimming. She competed in her first Olympics at the age of 14, and is more recently the author of "In the Water They Can't See You Cry: A Memoir".[9] In this memoir as well as in recent interviews, Beard opens up about her experience with bulimia nervosa. Newspaper reviews commented on Beard's weight as she went through puberty in the public eye, and she developed a goal to become thinner. In college, she was throwing up six to seven times a day, was exhausted all of the time, and was still very self-conscious about her body. She revealed in a speech at Cal Poly San Luis Obispo that she cared more about being thin than her swimming performance.[10] While Beard still struggles with self-image today, she has recovered with the support of her husband and is now helping to educate others about the risks of eating disorders.

There are a plethora of athletes who have advocated for positive body image in sports. Kayla Harrison is an Olympic Champion in judo, a sport that often promotes the idea that the lighter an athlete is, the better they will perform. Harrison argues against this mentality, as she doesn't cut weight and tries to promote that strong is beautiful.[11] Serena Williams is one of the most famous tennis players of all time and has won 73 single championships. Even with this success, Williams has faced scrutiny about her body as well, including comments that she looks like a man. In response Williams has stated, "I'm not asking you to like my body. I'm just asking you to let me be me. Because I'm going to influence a girl who does look like me, and I want her to feel good about herself".[12] Simone Biles won four gold medals in gymnastics at the 2016 Olympics and is considered one of the most successful gymnasts of all time. But she also faced criticism of her physique and was often bullied at school for her build. Biles promotes positive self-image as well, and told CNN, "You can judge my body all you want, but at the end of the day it's MY body. I love it and I'm comfortable in my skin".[13] Struggles with body image are thus a very prominent issue in athletics today.

As disordered eating and sufficient caloric intake are issues that influence athletes of many sports at all levels, different diagnoses have been developed to help identify these issues in athletes. In 1993, the American College of Sports Medicine defined the concept of the Female Athlete Triad as a first step.[14] The Female Athlete Triad is a condition that involves reduced energy/disordered eating, menstruation changes, and low bone mineral density. Athletes that have the Female Athlete Triad have symptoms that lie on a spectrum from completely healthy to amenorrhea, osteoporosis, and low energy. In 2007, the IOC redefined the Female Athlete Triad as Relative Energy Deficiency in Sport (RED-S) after conducting more research that revealed that the symptoms are more of a syndrome than a triad. RED-S is defined as a syndrome that results from energy deficiency and can influence metabolic rate, menstruation, bone health, immunity, protein synthesis, and cardiovascular and psychological health. There are short- and long-term impacts of RED-S, including nutrient deficiencies, fatigue, decreased athletic performance, medical complications, bone loss, changes in bone structure, and mental health decline. The change from the Female Athlete Triad to RED-S is a recent one, but this broader definition helps to accurately identify the syndrome in athletes and provide help.[15]

PREVIOUS PREVENTION PROJECTS

Disordered eating and RED-S are issues in the general population, but they disproportionately influence female athletes. However, the prevalence of such conditions has been shown to be decreased with intervention and education. Different programs have been implemented in the past in order to help address the issues of disordered eating and RED-S (or Female Athlete Triad at the time). SPRING Forward Girls is a program that has learned from these past examples and is striving for future progress.

The Body Project was one of the first projects that aimed to promote body acceptance and prevent eating disorders among adolescent and young girls. The methods of this program were published in 2007 and were designed and evaluated at Stanford University; Trinity University in San Antonio, Texas; Trinity College, Hartford Connecticut; University of South Florida; Iowa State University; and Yale University. The Body Project had the goal of reducing current and future disordered eating. The main approach that the Body Project implemented was having participants use cognitive dissonance. In this approach, the girls and athletes voluntarily argued against concepts such as society's pressure to be thin, which in turn reduced behavior that follows this ideal and the risks of eating disorders that come with it. The Body Project involved written, verbal, and behavioral exercises and focused on the participants, rather than the leaders, critiquing the thin ideal to yield best results. When participants voluntarily critique the societal pressure to be thin through the activities of the program, there is an inconsistency between their actions and their critiques. This causes them to change their behavior and leads to a reduction of body dissatisfaction, unhealthy dieting, and eating disorders. The Body Project implemented this idea of cognitive dissonance through interactive sessions, having the participants practice the learned skills in exercises, applying the skills learned through homework, using motivational enhancement exercises to increase participation, and holding group activities to create a supportive environment. While this program was targeted toward female athletes that were at risk for developing eating disorders, it was shown to be effective in non–high-risk populations as well. The Body Project was implemented across many different labs and found consistently to reduce eating disorders and promote body positivity, as well as outperform other interventions of the time.[16]

In 2019, research on the efficacy of the Female Athlete Body Project was published. The Female Athlete Body Project is a behavioral eating disorder risk factor reduction program that targets collegiate female athletes and is based on healthy weight intervention. This program focused on healthy weight intervention as opposed to dissonance intervention as new research revealed that although both methods produced similar results, participants preferred the healthy eating focus.[17] The Female Athlete Body Project focuses on reducing eating disorder symptoms and risk factors, but also acknowledges that eating disorder cases are often closely linked to the Female Athlete Triad (now known as RED-S). The Female Athlete Body Project involves participants attending one peer-led session per week for a period of three weeks. In these sessions participants would learn to strive for what the program refers to as the athlete-specific healthy ideal, which is defined as the way an athlete's body looks when they are striving for maximum physical and mental health, quality of life, and athletic performance. This process included identifying differences between the healthy ideal and society and sport-specific ideals, learning about the Female Athlete Triad, nutrition, goal setting, body image exercises, how to balance caloric intake and use, and sleep. The nutritional information given was not sport specific, but rather focused on nutrient density and healthy eating. Some of the activities included practicing responding to overhead "fat talk", as well as writing a letter to a younger athlete encouraging her to strive for a healthy ideal. The Female Athlete Body Project found there was a decrease in thin-ideal internalization among those who participated. This project demonstrated that a short intervention could have significant impacts on eating-disorder symptoms and risk factors through 18 months after the sessions. The Female Athlete Body Project thus is a beneficial program that is still being used in collegiate programs to promote body positivity, reduce eating disorder risks and symptoms, and educate about RED-S.[18]

SPRING Forward Girls is a program that has learned from previous initiatives' success and methods and is expanding the impact. SPRING stands for Strength and Positivity Rooted in Nutrition for Girls. Previous programs such as the Body Project and the Female Athlete Body Project have had success at reducing eating disorder risks and increasing body positivity among female college athletes. But these issues do not solely exist at the collegiate level. SPRING Forward Girls aims to implement the findings of these programs at the high school level. High school female athletes, often beginning to become more serious in their sports, are also vulnerable to body issue problems as their bodies are changing and they are feeling societal pressures. This program hopes to intervene at this young age to prevent the onset of eating disorders and RED-S in high school, or later if athletes elect to participate in college sports. SPRING Forward Girls involve three, one-hour long sessions that are spread throughout the athlete's season, with the first session when the season begins and the last before a big end-of-season competition. Like the Female Athlete Body Project, this program focuses on teaching the athletes about the differences between societal and sport-specific ideals and a healthy athlete body ideal. SPRING Forward Girls also educates about healthy eating by providing information about the importance of nutrition as well as the impacts and causes of RED-S. Sessions involve splitting the girls up into smaller groups to promote participation and connection, and there are activities with handouts, group discussions, and small homework assignments to apply what was learned. SPRING Forward Girls has a goal of reducing disordered eating, educating about RED-S, and increasing body positivity in high-school female athletes both now and in the future.

Notably, although this started with high school athletes, some of the athletes who underwent the program are now utilizing the teaching at their collegiate clubs and teams. So, this book does include some instruction for implementation beyond the adolescent years.

AN ATHLETE'S STORY: Mia

As a high schooler, running was a reservoir of all things positive for me—a stress reliever after school, a way to make new friends, and something I seemed to naturally excel at. I never really thought of running as surrounded by my perceptions of eating. I ate when I was hungry and didn't stop until I was full.

When I made it to the collegiate level in cross country/track and field, I believed all my hard work and dreams were finally falling into place. I was willing to do whatever it took to reach the national level and fulfill my potential. I trusted the staff at my school, and most of all, I trusted my coach.

I came to realize my coach had a true "win-at-all-costs" mindset, and because of this, I quickly overtrained and developed a femoral stress fracture. Now, rather than evaluate the rapid increase in training I had undergone, my weight was targeted instead. I was put on a restrictive diet by the department's nutritionist, isolated from my team to do specific, weight-loss workouts with the strength coach, and given a weight-loss book as a spring break "gift".

I have never been an individual lacking in personal body confidence, but it hurts to progressively limit your meals prior to weekly weigh-ins with the nutritionist in order to look like you lost weight. It hurts to have a coach tell you that you are doing personalized workouts because you are "a little chubby". It hurts to be told the reason you have recurrent injuries is because your skeletal system simply cannot handle all the excess fat on your body (mind you I was told by a physician prior to this that I was actually underweight).

This was all before I even finished my first year of collegiate running. Because conversation was so stigmatized surrounding this issue, I thought I was the only one being told to lose weight—I internalized everything I was told and began to develop an incredibly unhealthy relationship with my body.

My running career was defined by constant injuries, and each time, my weight was placed as the culprit. As if it wasn't difficult enough to be injured and removed from what I loved, I then knew I would have to undergo a personal attack on my diet, only alienating myself even more from a healthy perception of my body.

Running was no longer just a stress reliever and fun with my teammates—I began to calculate how long each run needed to be to in order to ensure I could still eat while not gaining any weight. I picked my body apart when I looked in the mirror. If I was not noticeably toned, then I was disgusted with my body.

All this reached a pivot during the spring of my junior year—I began to have significant gastrointestinal problems, which limited my ability to eat before training. I skipped meals each day in order to ensure I could avoid issues during practice. This led to significant weight loss (12–15 pounds in the span of 3 months)—one of the few times during my collegiate career that my coach actually appreciated the way my body looked.

I eventually discovered I had Crohn's disease along with a diagnosis of RED-S. I began an appropriate treatment plan—which also included gaining weight. This is where my coach felt he had to intervene and called me in for a meeting.

What you have to understand is that my coach knew it was wrong to discuss an athlete's weight, but of course, there are ways to get around every rule. Rather my coach told me that I was doing every piece of training correct—except for one tiny factor. A factor he could not discuss with me but which he could tell me had to do with my recent medical advice and decisions regarding nutrition. Well, I think I can put that one together. Upon discussion with other staff members, my suspicions were confirmed. My coach felt I had to maintain the same weight as when I had uncontrolled Crohn's disease in order to run well—the main factor to ensure athletic performance in his eyes.

This was the point I decided I was done and could no longer represent an institution and coach with such twisted ideals. I forwent my fifth year of eligibility and have since spent my time advocating for awareness regarding this issue.

I am proud of myself for leaving such a toxic coaching environment and realizing I deserve better. I want to make it clear, however, that you cannot just leave a program like this and also immediately remove the cruel words and actions of ignorant staff members. Redevelopment of a healthy relationship with your body takes time, but it absolutely can be done and is worth it.

I urge coaches and athletic staff to understand the effects of their words and actions surrounding athletes' bodies. I ask physicians and other medical professionals to watch vigilantly for signs of disordered eating and body dysmorphia within the young athletes they treat. I ask family members and teammates to recognize the red flags and reach out to those struggling. And most of all, I ask you, the one reading this book right now, to be a voice in this message—to be the individual who changes the culture surrounding eating and body image within your own school or athletic program.

When I was in the midst of struggling with my own body image, I thought I was the only one—be loud regarding this issue because you do not know who is listening and who is reaching for your help. Let's be the ones to change the conversation surrounding eating and body image within sport because our voices and this problem do matter.

CITATIONS

1. Astor, Maggie. "A Gymnast's Death Was Supposed to Be a Wake Up Call. What Took So Long?" *New York Times*, April 26, 2022. Updated April 28, 2002.
2. Cain, Mary. "I Was the Fastest Girl in America, Until I Joined Nike." *New York Times*, November 7, 2019.
3. Futterman, Matthew. "Another of Alberto Salazar's Runners Says He Ridiculed Her Body for Years." *New York Times*, November 14, 2019.
4. Goucher, Kara. "Eat a Dorito." By FloTrack, April 21, 2007.
5. Strout, Erin. "Kara Goucher on Alberto Salazar's Doping Violations Ban: 'I Feel at Peace'." *Women's Running*, October 6, 2019.
6. Ackerman, Kathryn, Trent Stellingwerff, Kirsty Elliot-Sale, Amy Baltzell, Mary Cain, Kara Goucher, Lauren Fleshman, and Margo Mountjoy. "#REDS (Relative Energy Deficiency in Sport): Time for a Revolution in Sports Culture and Systems to Improve Athlete Health and Performance." *PubMed*, January 10, 2020.
7. Crouse, Karen. "Gracie Gold's Battle for Olympic Glory Ended in a Fight to Save Herself." *New York Times*, January 25, 2019.
8. "Olympic Skating Champion Lipnitskaya Opens Up about Anorexia." *Associated Press*, September 12, 2017 https://apnews.com/article/395db10682a04d2cac073ae37569d3fc
9. Howard, Courtney. "Inside the Summer Olympics: Competitive Swimming & Eating Disorders." *Eating Disorder Hope*. Accessed November 22, 2020. https://www.eatingdisorderhope.com/blog/inside-summer-olympics-competitive-swimming-eating-disorders
10. Koschalk, Katie. "Olympic Swimmer Addresses Eating Disorders." *Mustang News*, November 18, 2009. https://mustangnews.net/olympic-swimmer-addresses-eating-disorders/
11. Glock, Allison. "'No One Will Break Me': The Conversation with Jod Champion Kayla Harrison." *ESPN*, July 11, 2016. https://www.espn.com/espnw/voices/story/_/id/16998379/the-conversation-kayla-harrison-first-american-win-gold-olympic-judo
12. Kahn, Howie. "Serena Williams, Wonder Woman, Is Our September Cover." *Self*, August 1, 2016. https://www.self.com/story/serena-williams-september-cover-interview
13. Murphy, Chris, and Aleks Klosok. "Simone Biles: Body Image Issue Was Biggest Personal Challenge." *CNN*, July 7, 2017. https://www.cnn.com/2017/07/03/sport/simone-biles-olympics-rio-2016-body-image/index.html

14. American College of Sports Medicine. "The Female Athlete Triad: Disordered Eating, Amenorrhea, Osteoporosis—A Call to Action." *Sports Med Bull*, 1992, 27:4.
15. Mountjoy, Marog, Jorunn Sundgot-Borgen, Louise Burke, Susan Carter, Naama Constantini, Constance Lebrun, Nanna Meyer, Roberta Sherman, Kathrin Steffen, Richard Budgett, and Arne Ljungqvist. "The IOC Consensus Statement: Beyond the Female Athlete Triad—Relative Energy Deficiency in Sport (RED-S)." *British Journal of Sports Medicine*, February 3, 2014.
16. Strice, Eric. *The Body Project*. New York: Oxford University Press, 2007.
17. Becker, Carolyn, Leda McDaniel, Stephanie Bull, Marc Powell, and Kevin McIntyre. "Can We Reduce Eating Disorder Risk Factors in Female College Athletes? A Randomized Exploratory Investigation of Two Peer-Led Interventions." *PubMed*, October 22, 2011.
18. Stewart, Tiffany, Tarryn Pollard, Tom Hilderbrandt, Nicole Wesley, Lisa Kilpela, and Carolyn Becker. "The Female Athlete Body Project Study: 18-Month Outcomes in Eating Disorder Symptoms and Risk Factors." *US National Library of Medicine*, July 17, 2019.

2 Nutritional Needs of Adolescent Female Athletes

Andrew Dole
University of Waikato, Hamilton, New Zealand

Kathryn Vidlock
Rocky Vista University, Parker, CO, USA

Catherine Liggett
University of Colorado School of Medicine, Aurora, CO, USA

CONTENTS

DOI: 10.1201/b23228-2

WORDS TO KNOW

ADOLESCENT ATHLETE   Refers to all athletes, male and female, between the ages of 12–18. Teen or teenage is not a term used to differentiate athletes.[1] The age of 18 is adulthood by social means, not biological.

AMENORRHEA   The term used for not having or missing periods; the loss of menses.

AMINO ACIDS   The small units that create a complete protein. There are 9 essential and 11 non-essential amino acid that make up the 20 that the body uses.

BRANCH CHAIN AMINO ACIDS   The three essential amino acids leucine, isoleucine, and valine. Of all the amino acids they are the most responsible for protein synthesis and anabolism.

CARBOHYDRATE (CHO)   Dietary energy source that contains 4 calories/g. Fiber, sugar, simple, complex, and starchy are familiar CHO types. Food examples: rice, bread, pasta, potato, sugar, oatmeal, fruits, vegetables, soda, candy.

COMPLEMENTARY PROTEINS   The combination of two or more incomplete proteins to create a complete protein. Examples would be beans and rice or peanut butter and bread.

COMPLETE PROTEINS   Foods or supplements that contain all nine of the essential amino acids. All animal proteins are complete.

DISACCHARIDE   A sugar made of two simple sugars and can be broken into the single smaller monosaccharides.

ENERGY   A nutrition term that refers to the ability to do work. Our body converts food to calories the unit of energy used by the body to do "work".

ENERGY AVAILABILITY   Calories eaten (minus) calorie needs for sport = available energy for body function.

ESSENTIAL AMINO ACIDS   Must be obtained from food because the body cannot create enough to meet the body's demands.

ESSENTIAL FATTY ACIDS   The omega-3 and omega-6 fatty acids that the body cannot produce enough of and must be obtained from food.

FAT A dietary energy source that contains 9 calories/g. Monounsaturated, polyunsaturated, saturated, and trans-fat are common food-related terms. Food examples: olive oil, peanuts, vegetable oil, lard, butter.

FOLLICULAR PHASE Starts on first day of period and ends at ovulation.

INCOMPLETE PROTEINS Do not contain all nine of the essential amino acids and cannot be used to form a protein unit. Most all plant proteins are incomplete.

KCAL Short for kilocalorie; a measure of the energy available in a food. Our body converts food into energy and it is measured in kcals. It is common to just use the word "calorie" in non-science or health fields; food labels for example use the word *calorie* instead of kcal or kilocalorie.

KILOGRAM (kg) 2.2 pounds. To calculate kg from pounds do the following: weight in pounds divided by 2.2. For example 130#/2.2 = 59 kg.

LUTEAL PHASE Days after ovulation up to start of period.

MACRONUTRIENTS The nutrients protein, fat, and carbohydrates that are needed in large amounts and often measured in grams, ounces, or pounds.

MENARCHE The first menstrual cycle a female experiences. Average age this occurs is 12.5 years.

MICRONUTRIENTS Include vitamins and minerals. These are required in small amounts and are measured in much smaller units: microgram, milligram, and international units (IU).

MONOSACCHARIDE A sugar that cannot be broken down into smaller units.

MONOUNSATURATED FAT Contains a double bond, which reduces the number of hydrogens. Example: $CH_3-CH_2-CH = CH-CH_2-CH_3$ (12 hydrogens).

OMEGA-3 Consist of ALA, EPA, and DHA acids found in fish, seafood, seaweed, nuts, and seeds.

OMEGA-6 Polyunsaturated fat found in tofu, eggs, nuts, seeds, and vegetable oils.

POLYSACCHARIDE A large starch made of simple sugars that can be broken down into many monosaccharides.

POLYUNSATURED FAT Contains two or more double bonds, reducing the number of hydrogens. Example: $CH_3-CH=C=C-CH-CH_3$ (8 hydrogens).

PROTEIN (PRO) Dietary source of energy and amino acids that contains 4 calories/g. Found in plant and animal foods. Food examples: chicken, beef, pork, nuts, fish, quinoa, soy, milk, cheese, yogurt, whey.

SATURATED FAT Full of hydrogen bonds, hence the term saturated. Example: $CH_3-CH_2-CH_2-CH_2-CH_2-CH_3$ (14 hydrogens).

TRANS-FAT A liquid plant-based oil with hydrogens added to create a solid fat similar to animal saturated fats. The hydrogen density is greater than natural saturated fats.

WHAT ARE THE ENERGY (CALORIC) NEEDS OF A YOUNG FEMALE ATHLETE?

There are no calorie calculators for the adolescent (12–18-year-old) athlete. All current recommendations for how much a young athlete should eat every day are based on general health guidelines for growth and development. It's difficult to account for hormone changes, puberty, and growth needs of young athletic human. Adding exercise to the equation, especially different forms of exercise, just makes things more complicated.

What recommendations do exist are based on the Schofield equation to determine the amount of energy needed when doing nothing; lying in bed for example. This is known as resting energy expenditure (REE). REE is then multiplied by an activity factor (AF) that represents how much activity will be done in a day: school, sports practice, homework. REE × AF = is just an estimate of how much to eat. Many things affect this basic math equation that cannot be accounted for, including quantity of muscle mass, hormones, sex, fat, puberty, and how much food is eaten daily.[1]

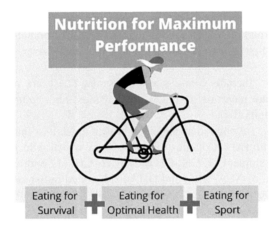

The best we can do now is estimate energy needs for the young athlete. We cannot put an exact number to the calories needed each day, but we can use measurable markers of failure or insufficiency to catch slip-ups in fueling the adolescent athlete at very early stages. This is where the adult support system can and must do better.

WHAT ABOUT PROTEIN? (PROTEIN NEEDS)

Dietary reference ranges, such as the RDA (recommended daily allowance) prevent deficiencies. They do not account for active lifestyles and may not be optimal for basic growth and development needs. For example, protein needs in females and males, ages 12–18, is 0.8 g/kg a day. However, multiple studies show that 1.2–1.8 g/kg/d is required to maintain and rebuild tissue in active adolescents; a significant 50–125% difference from the recommended daily value of 0.8 g/kg. During the follicular phase of the menstrual cycle, athletes likely need a little more protein.[2] The American College of Sports Medicine recommends 1.2 g/kg/d to 2.0 g/kg/d distributed evenly throughout the month because it is more consistent and easy to follow.[3]

20 GRAMS OF PROTEIN

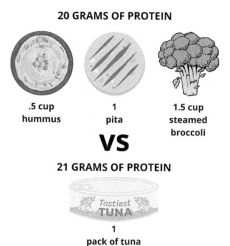

.5 cup
hummus

1
pita

1.5 cup
steamed
broccoli

VS

21 GRAMS OF PROTEIN

1
pack of tuna

To meet these increased protein needs the following best practices are suggested:

- Eat 15–25 g of protein at each meal. Total amount differs per athlete needs and is based on weight.
- Time a protein-based meal within one hour after training or an event.
- Eat protein meals every 3–5 hours throughout the day.

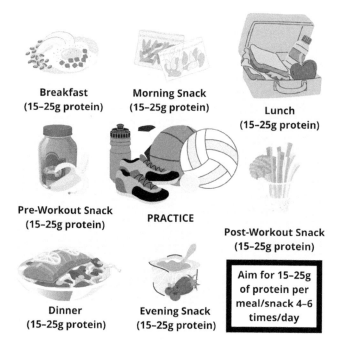

Breakfast
(15–25g protein)

Morning Snack
(15–25g protein)

Lunch
(15–25g protein)

Pre-Workout Snack
(15–25g protein)

PRACTICE

Post-Workout Snack
(15–25g protein)

Dinner
(15–25g protein)

Evening Snack
(15–25g protein)

Aim for 15–25g
of protein per
meal/snack 4–6
times/day

PROTEIN GENERAL INFORMATION

- The building blocks of the human body and a protected nutrient, dietary protein is so important the body does not burn it as an energy source except in dire situations of starvation, massive injury, disease (cancer), or incredible metabolic demands with lack of adequate fuel sources.
- Essential amino acids and proteins are key nutrients for several reasons. The most well-known function of protein is the repair and creation of tissue and muscle. A lesser-known protein role is turning on and off genetic signals within DNA, as enzymes for chemical reactions like digestion, creation of antibodies for the immune system, hormone production, cell signaling, and of course the structure of cells, tissues, and organs.

AMINO ACIDS

- Proteins are made up of thousands of smaller units called amino acids. There are two types of amino acids: essential and non-essential. Both types are required but non-essential can be produced in the body, unlike essential amino acids that must be obtained from food. Among the essential amino acids are three with the strongest protein-building potential. They are called the branch-chained amino acids: valine, leucine, and isoleucine.

Non-Essential Amino Acids	Essential Amino Acids
Very much required but body can make what is needed	Body cannot produce what is needed so must get from food
Alanine Arginine Asparagine Aspartic Acid Cysteine Glutamic Acid Glutamine Glycine Proline Serine Tyrosine	Histidine Lysine Methionine Phenylalanine Threonine Tryptophan Branched Chain (BCAA): Valine Isoleucine Leucine

COMPLETE AND INCOMPLETE PROTEINS

- Not all foods provide essential amino acids. Proteins from animals are called complete proteins. They have all nine essential amino acids and when eaten provide all the amino acids required to create new protein. Most plant proteins are incomplete proteins, meaning they are missing or very low in one or more of the essential amino acids. By themselves they would be unable to create new protein.
- There are exceptions. Some plants are complete, providing adequate amounts of the essential amino acids just like animal products: quinoa, buckwheat, hempseed, blue-green algae, soy, and chia.
- Is there a concern for protein deficiency in vegan athletes? Realistically, yes, but not because of incomplete proteins. For example, eating a wide variety of plants each day easily provides all nine of the essential amino acids. It's the concept of complimentary proteins—two incomplete protein foods paired together create a complete protein.
- Grains are low in lysine. Beans and nuts are low in methionine. Eat them together and the problem is solved. A peanut butter and jelly sandwich, for example (bread and nuts).

There are many complete protein pairings for plant foods.

- Beans and rice
- Hummus and bread
- Noodles and peanut sauce
- Lentils and rice
- Greens and seeds
- Oatmeal and nuts

The risk for protein deficiency without animal products comes in two forms. First is the volume of food required to obtain sufficient daily protein needs. Except for soy, plant foods do not provide the same protein density as animal sources. Fullness is an obstacle. Female athletes may already be body conscious. Feeling full and eating large amounts of food will not come naturally. Additionally, with the volume of plant food required, potential issues with the associated fiber intake such as gaseousness and GI distress exist. Access is another barrier. It can be difficult for a young athlete to have access to food throughout the day, highlighting the importance of convenient nutrient-dense meals.

To obtain 20 g of protein from hummus, pita, and greens: combine 0.5 cup hummus, 1 pita, 1.5 cups steamed broccoli at 456 calories, 20 g PRO, 67 g CHO, and 13 g FAT vs 1 pouch of tuna at 21 g PRO.

- There is a lack of food knowledge to replace what has been omitted. An example would be increasing soy and quinoa to make up for the absence of dairy and meat. It's quite common for young athletes and adults to remove entire food groups from their diet without replacing them. As mentioned, not all foods provide the same nutrients and more food maybe required.

WHICH IS BETTER?

The plant-based version of the preceding example solves many female athlete nutrition problems. It's high in carbohydrates, rich in vitamins, minerals, and phytochemicals, and provides more calories to achieve the same protein goals. Female athletes notoriously underconsume calories, carbohydrates, protein, and food in general. But cost, consistency, time, and energy can be obstacles to making more complicated meals. Is it likely that the athlete will have access to and then eat all the required food consistently enough?

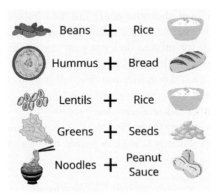

CARBOHYDRATES

WHAT IS THE CARBOHYDRATE NEED OF A YOUNG FEMALE ATHLETE?

The primary fuel source for athletes are carbohydrates (CHO). Whether the sport is endurance, power, or speed, a type of sugar, primarily glucose and fructose, fuels performance. Fat, fat adaption, and sex differences in nutrient use do exist beyond puberty, but the importance of CHO in performance is not lessened. The carbohydrate (CHO) guidelines are based on adults with no age-appropriate research. What research does exist tells us that adolescents and adults use carbohydrates the same way and that their fueling needs for sport are similar.[1] However, the differences in athlete body size and training loads between adolescents and adults do need be accounted for. This can be done by following well-established guidelines for CHO intake.

> *CHO Needs Daily* low-intensity or skill-based activity: 3–5 g/kg/d; moderate exercise program (e.g., training 1 h/d): 5–7 g/kg/d; endurance program (e.g., training 1–3 h/d): 6–10 g/kg/d; extreme exercise program (e.g., training 4–5 h/d) 8–12 g/kg/d.
>
> *CHO Needs during Training/Event* short duration (0–45 min): None required; sustained high intensity (45–75 min): small amounts 15–30 g, typically part of a sports drink; medium/long duration (75 min–2.5 h): 30–60 g/h; extended durations (more than 2.5 h): CHO intake per hour based on the most the athlete can tolerate.
>
> *CHO Needs Two Sessions per Day* less than 8 h between sessions: 1–1.2 g/kg/h for first 4 h, followed by regular meals.

Carbohydrates—The Basics

There are three main fuel sources for the body: carbohydrates, fat, and the creatine phosphate system. Each has a purpose and all three get used at the same time. How much of each gets used depends on the intensity of what the body is doing.

Think of creatine phosphate as the lightning fuel of the body. It's incredibly fast but limited to about 8–10 seconds of work. Fat is slow burning, like big logs on a fire. There are days of fuel stored and when it's burning it lasts a long time, but it's hard to use in a hurry. Carbohydrates are the middle ground, with about 2 h of storage. They burn efficiently and can be used quickly. Of the three energy sources, during moderate to intense exercise, carbohydrates are the preferred energy: the body uses a higher percentage of them to fuel work.

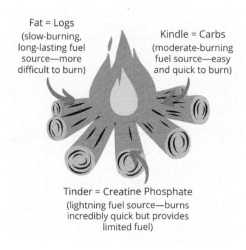

Fat = Logs
(slow-burning, long-lasting fuel source—more difficult to burn)

Kindle = Carbs
(moderate-burning fuel source—easy and quick to burn)

Tinder = Creatine Phosphate
(lightning fuel source—burns incredibly quick but provides limited fuel)

Carbohydrates are also macronutrients and provide 4 kcals/g. They are needed in large amounts and often measured in grams, ounces, or pounds. Alcohol and water have been added to this list because they also are measured in large units.

Carbohydrate	1g = 4 kcals
Protein	1g = 4 kcals
Fat	1g = 9 kcals
Alcohol	1g = 7 kcals
Water	1g = 0 kcals

SCIENCEY DETAILS

It is glucose that fuels the body and glucose is a carbohydrate. The body breaks down the carbohydrates we eat and turns them into glucose. Glucose is then stored in two different forms: glycogen and fat. Glycogen can be found in the liver and the muscles. Muscle glycogen can only be used by the muscles. It cannot be released into the body to regulate blood sugar. However, liver glycogen can do both. It can be released into the bloodstream to regulate blood sugar or be transported to working muscles for fuel.

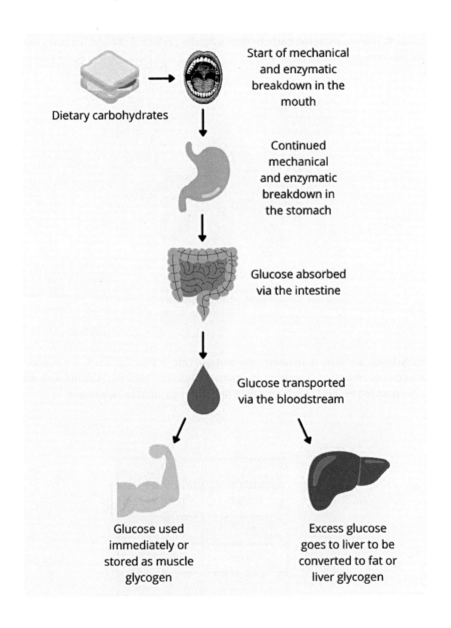

IMPORTANCE OF CARBOHYDRATES

Carbohydrates are more than just an exercise fuel. Many body functions rely on carbohydrates, including

- Fuel brain and neuron cells, which rely almost exclusively on glucose from liver for energy.
- Maintain blood glucose levels.
  - Mental and physical performance.
  - Appetite control.
- Spare proteins from being burned as energy.
  - Muscle wasting.
- Necessary for the complete use of fat as fuel.
  - Oxidation of fat.
- Maintain blood pH.
  - Prevents ketoacidosis (body producing ketones when there is not enough available glucose accessible for cell use).
    - Blood pH imbalance from a buildup of fat oxidation by-product.

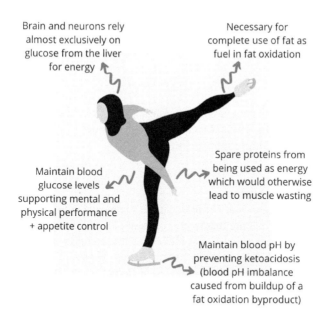

TYPES OF CARBOHYDRATES

The foods we eat provide simple and complex carbohydrates. At the end of the day, both get broken down into glucose. Complex carbohydrates just take longer. Simple carbohydrates are sugars. They come in two forms: monosaccharides and disaccharides. *Mono* is a prefix that means one, *di* is a prefix that means two, and *poly* is a prefix meaning many. Sugars digest quickly because they have lots of branches, making it easy to break down.

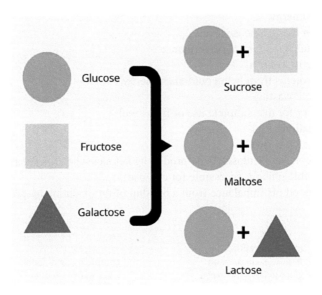

Complex carbohydrates are starch. A starch is polysaccharide made of sugars in a massive chain, but with fewer branches. They are harder to digest because break-down can't occur at multiple spots in the chain.

Sources of Carbohydrates

Most whole foods are a mixture of both simple sugars and complex starches. Nearly all the lists on the internet are incorrect. For example, white rice, bananas, potatoes, and white bread contain starch. That makes them a complex carbohydrate, but on many sites they are listed as simple carbohydrates. However, some carbohydrates are more complex than others because of their fiber content. Brown rice or a high-fiber bread would be good examples. The least confusing are the pure simple sugars. Examples are honey, table sugar (sucrose), maple syrup, corn syrup, brown rice syrup, agave, fructose from fruit juices, and sports products like gels, maltodextrin, and sports drinks.

A good message here is to look at the food labels for at least two things:

1. Total sugars
2. Added sugars

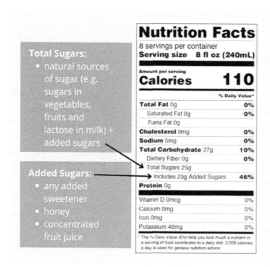

No processed food is truly safe from added sugar, but food labels as of 2020–2021 are required to list "added sugars". Naturally occurring sugars found in vegetables, fruits, and lactose in milk are not viewed as added sugars. However, any sweetener added to a product, even honey and concentrated fruit sugars, are considered an added sugar.

Lastly, an athlete needs both simple and complex carbohydrates. You can't eat a bowl of brown rice during practice, games, or events. It's too slow to digest and would cause serious stomach upset. On the other hand, drinking soda with a bag of gummy bears isn't quality nutrition for lunch each day.

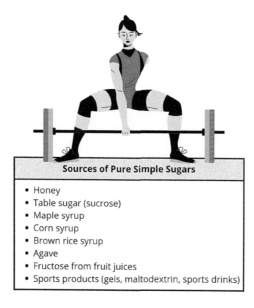

Sources of Pure Simple Sugars

- Honey
- Table sugar (sucrose)
- Maple syrup
- Corn syrup
- Brown rice syrup
- Agave
- Fructose from fruit juices
- Sports products (gels, maltodextrin, sports drinks)

IS FAT GOOD OR BAD? (FAT NEEDS)

Fat is important. It is required for hormone production, growth and development, and many other functions within the body. It is also an important energy source for life and sport. There are 9 calories in every 1 g of fat. Compared to 4 calories per 1 g of protein or carbohydrates this dense energy source is valuable in meeting daily energy goals. It can also be used to meet energy needs in athletes who have difficulty eating enough every day.

About 20–35% of the total calories in a day should come from healthy fats such as nuts, avocado, and fish, and oils like olive, canola, or avocado. Saturated fat should be limited to less than 10%.[1] Saturated fat sources come from animal meats, coconut, dairy, and processed or fried foods.

Eating by percentages isn't effective and recommendations like 20–35% need to be translated to the food athletes will eat. Training plates are good visual teaching aides that help athletes understand how to choose the best types of foods to meet their fueling needs. Examples of training plates and learning tools are provided in a separate chapter.

DIETARY FATS

Like other macronutrients, fat does so much more than just provide fat for our body. It helps in cushioning organs, blood clotting, vitamin absorption, hormone productions, wound healing, and maintaining cell walls.

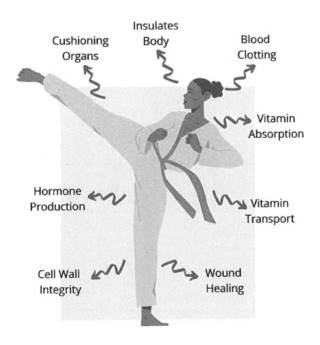

There are two main types of fat: saturated and unsaturated. The difference between these fats is quite simple. Saturated fats have the maximum number of hydrogens the chemical bonds can hold. Sounds complicated, but it isn't. When a sponge is saturated it cannot hold anymore. The same is true for a saturated fat. It's full of hydrogens. Unsaturated fats come in two types: monounsaturated and polyunsaturated. They are different because they have fewer hydrogens.

Examples:

- Saturated fat: $CH_3-CH_2-CH_2-CH_2-CH_2-CH_3$ (14 hydrogens)
- Monounsaturated fat: $CH_3-CH_2-CH = CH-CH_2-CH_3$ (12 hydrogens)
- Polyunsaturated: $CH_3-CH=C=C-CH-CH_3$ (8 hydrogens)

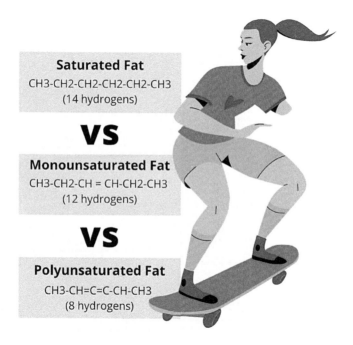

CHOLESTEROL AND HYDROGENS

Why do hydrogens matter? The body produces most of its cholesterol from hydrogens. The more hydrogens available the more cholesterol it will make. A diet high in saturated fat and sugar will usually result in high total cholesterol levels.

What is cholesterol? Cholesterol is an important steroid produced in the body. It is necessary to create sex hormones, vitamin D, cell membranes, brain signaling, and food digestion enzymes. There are two forms of cholesterol: low-density (LDL) and high-density (HDL) lipoproteins. LDL transports cholesterol to where it's needed in the body. HDL transports excess cholesterol in the body back to the liver to be reprocessed. Cholesterol, especially LDL gets a bad rap, but it's 100% necessary to be alive.

LDL comes in two different forms, light and fluffy or dense. It is believed that dense LDL cholesterol contributes to cardiovascular disease. However, there is a lack of cause and effect, meaning there is no proof that cholesterol itself is a direct cause. Other factors such as lifestyle, genetics, age, and illnesses are part of the equation in addition to cholesterol. Although when trying to lower cholesterol, the first step is always reducing saturated fat and sugar sources in the diet.

Sugar can cause high cholesterol—especially from high fructose corn syrup. Excess calories from sugar are taken to the liver and made into fatty acids, which increase the amount of dense LDL. So, what is worse for cardiovascular disease—sugar or saturated fat? Here are some facts,

Take a moment to reflect on the standard American diet: high in sugar, packaged foods with partially hydrogenated fats, soda, energy drinks, flavored coffees, high fructose corn syrups, etc.

Which should be limited?

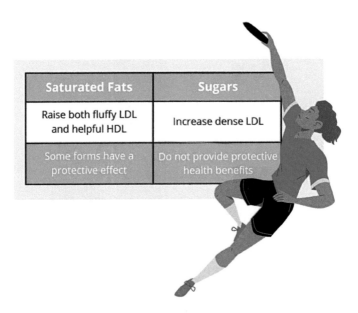

Saturated Fats	Sugars
Raise both fluffy LDL and helpful HDL	Increase dense LDL
Some forms have a protective effect	Do not provide protective health benefits

ESSENTIAL FATTY ACIDS—THE OMEGAS

Essential fatty acids cannot be made in sufficient quantities by the body and must be obtained from food or supplements. There are two types: omega-6 and omega-3. Omega-6 fatty acids are plentiful in most diets. They are used in maintaining bone health, metabolism, brain function, growth and development, gene activity, and cell development. Omega-3 fats come in three different forms: ALA, EPA, and DHA. Alpha linoleic acids (ALA) are found in plant foods and easily available in a diet rich with fruits and vegetables. ALA is used to create EPA and DHA as well as energy for the body to use. The process of converting ALA to EPA/DHA is very inefficient and not recommended as the only source of EPA/DHA. An example would be eating flaxseeds or walnuts, which are full of ALA, but would not provide much EPA/DHA.

Eicosapentaenoic acid (EPA) and docosahexaenoic acid (DHA) are found in animal foods and algae. They are the least abundant omega fats in most diets but have roles in major body systems: cardiovascular (heart), pulmonary (lung), immune, and endocrine (hormones) systems.

The media and pop culture knowledge around omega fats is based on inflammation. It is common to read that omega-6 fats are pro-inflammatory, while omega-3 fats are anti-inflammatory. This gives the impression of bad and good. This is not the case; both are necessary, and there is more to the story.

Omega-6 fats do not cause inflammation. They are building blocks to inflammation signaling, which is a good thing. Inflammation is required for healing and is very different than chronic inflammation. Think about when the body is cut or injured. The area around the injury swells. This swelling is a result of the body's protective and healing functions. When this protective effect persists for a long time (chronic) it is no longer helpful and becomes harmful to the body.

Omega-3 fats do not prevent or stop inflammation. They provide the building blocks for lessening inflammatory responses in body. Truthfully, science does not fully understand how omega fats work.

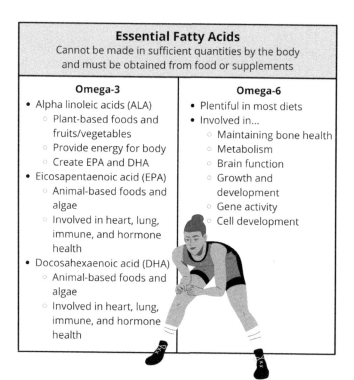

Essential Fatty Acids
Cannot be made in sufficient quantities by the body and must be obtained from food or supplements

Omega-3	Omega-6
• Alpha linoleic acids (ALA)	• Plentiful in most diets
○ Plant-based foods and fruits/vegetables	• Involved in...
○ Provide energy for body	○ Maintaining bone health
○ Create EPA and DHA	○ Metabolism
• Eicosapentaenoic acid (EPA)	○ Brain function
○ Animal-based foods and algae	○ Growth and development
○ Involved in heart, lung, immune, and hormone health	○ Gene activity
• Docosahexaenoic acid (DHA)	○ Cell development
○ Animal-based foods and algae	
○ Involved in heart, lung, immune, and hormone health	

SOURCES OF FATS

- Saturated—Animal meats, dairy, eggs, butter, baked goods, coconut oils, coconut milk
- Monounsaturated—Avocado, avocado oil, nuts, canola oil, olive oil
- Polyunsaturated—Seafood, vegetable oils, nuts, seeds
- Omega-3
- EPA: Fish, fish oil, fortified eggs, algae
- DHA: Flax, chia, walnuts, leafy greens, soy
- Trans—Any food that lists hydrogenated or partially hydrogenated oils (these are common in packaged foods especially: chips, baked goods, pastries, snack foods)

Saturated Fats	Monounsaturated Fats	Polyunsaturated Fats
• animal meats • dairy • eggs • butter • baked goods • coconut oil/milk	• avocado • avocado oil • nuts • canola oil • olive oil	• seafood • vegetable oils • nuts • seeds

Trans Fats	Omega-3 Fats	
	EPA	DHA

• food with hydrogenated or partially hydrogenated oils
• common in packaged foods
  ○ chips
  ○ baked goods
  ○ pastries
	• fish/fish oil
	• fortified eggs
	• algae
		• flax
		• chia
		• walnuts
		• leafy greens
		• soy

DOES NUTRITION CHANGE AFTER PUBERTY?

What Doesn't Change?

The menstrual cycle itself does not change nutrition needs drastically. Macronutrients like protein, carbohydrates, and fat as well as the total number of calories per day will not meaningfully change. Using the word "meaningfully" is purposeful because with menarche and the two phases of the menstrual cycle (follicular and luteal) there are changes to metabolism. For example, research shows that a growth spurt often precedes the first menstrual cycle. This growth spurt increases metabolism anywhere from 1–8 months before the first period and afterwards for about 1–4 months. An increase in calories, proteins, fats, vitamins, and minerals, for example, would all be based on the taller, heavier, human that just matured, and not so much the menstrual cycle. With every monthly cycle afterward there are ups and downs in energy metabolism based on the phase. However, recent research points out that the increased energy needs in the luteal phase are not actionable. This means that scientifically, yes there is a difference, but the change is so small it is not something that requires a nutrition or food change.

With young female athletes coming to terms with a menstrual cycle, the pressures of life, and the demands of sport, there are much bigger nutrition issues to worry about that impact health, well-being, and performance—for example, preventing chronic underfueling associated with female triad and RED-S by focusing efforts on eating enough food throughout every day. That is not to say that the menstrual cycle cannot be optimized with a little biohacking for the older female athlete once the main concerns are taken care of.

What Does Change?

Macronutrients may not change drastically because of the menstrual cycle, but one micronutrient does become a concern. The female athlete will need more iron once they begin having periods. However, it can't just be that simple. It's not just the menstrual cycle that matters. Factors such as diet choice and foods beliefs that limit food or omit food groups will also have major influence on micronutrient levels. Vegan and vegetarian diets have the greatest risk for nutrient deficiencies. Add all of that together and we still need to consider that athletes living at high altitude and those at an elite level of play may require more supervision from their healthcare team to ensure optimal intakes and avoid deficiencies from the higher level of training and competition.

IRON

Once a female starts menstruating, iron needs increase by 87%. Interestingly, most female athletes will not need more iron than their nonactive peers. There is a strong emphasis on consistently eating foods that provide iron and improve iron absorption. The recommended daily iron intake is 8 mg a day for premenstrual females, 15 mg a day for menstruating females, and 33 mg a day for vegetarians and vegans who are menstruating.[4,5]

Sources of Iron

- *Animal (4 heme iron)*
  - Beef, pork, chicken, tuna, turkey
- *Nonanimal (non-heme iron)*
  - Canned tomatoes, edamame, spinach, black beans, kidney beans, cashews, hummus, kale, potatoes, peas, lentils, tofu, fortified cereals

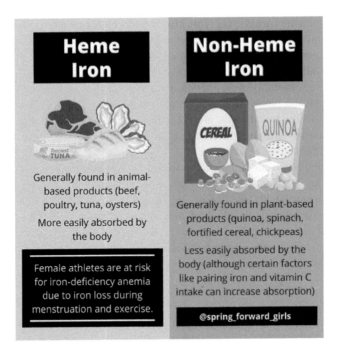

Heme Iron

Generally found in animal-based products (beef, poultry, tuna, oysters)

More easily absorbed by the body

Female athletes are at risk for iron-deficiency anemia due to iron loss during menstruation and exercise.

Non-Heme Iron

Generally found in plant-based products (quinoa, spinach, fortified cereal, chickpeas)

Less easily absorbed by the body (although certain factors like pairing iron and vitamin C intake can increase absorption)

@spring_forward_girls

Iron Absorption Concerns

Diets that exclude animal products need 1.8 times more iron daily because plant-based "non-heme" iron is not absorbed as well as animal iron sources. Also, phytates—a natural compound found in whole grains—and beans, the foundation of a non-meat diet—bind with iron and prevent absorption.

Iron Absorption Tips

- Eat a vitamin C source with meals. Vitamin C helps the absorption of iron.
- Drink green smoothies with leafy greens like spinach or kale made with orange juice or vitamin C–fortified juices.
- Visit with a provider for lab work. Supplementing iron without supervision is not recommended. Iron is extremely toxic and supplementation must be supervised.

CALCIUM

A lot of growth and development occurs between the ages of 13–18. The skeleton is very much a part of that growth process. In fact, the bone growth in adolescence matters for one's entire life. Poor bone health at early ages leads to high risk of a weakened bone structure (osteopenia) and severely weakened, brittle skeleton (osteoporosis). Hormones and nutrition both play a role in healthy bone development. Undereating daily leads to deficiencies in nutrients like calcium that are required to produce healthy bone structures. Additionally, estrogen is a key component of bone development. Chronic undereating causes irregular or missing periods, which decreases estrogen levels, which decreases bone mass development.

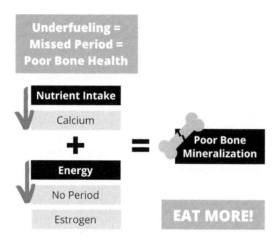

For females aged 9–18, the recommended daily allowance of calcium is 1300 mg/day. For adult women, the daily allowance is 1000 mg/day; for women over 50 the amount is 1200 mg/day.

High Calcium Per Serving Foods	Serving Size	mg/serving
Yogurt, plain, low fat	8 ounces	415
Orange juice, calcium fortified	1 cup	349
Mozzarella, part skim	1.5 ounces	333
Sardines, canned in oil, with bones	3 ounces	325
Cheddar cheese	1.5 ounces	307
Milk, nonfat	1 cup	299
Soy milk, calcium fortified	1 cup	299
Milk, reduced fat (2% milk fat)	1 cup	293
Yogurt, fruit, low fat	6 ounces	258
Tofu, firm, made with calcium sulfate	.5 cup	253
Cottage cheese, 1% milk fat	1 cup	138
Tofu, soft, made with calcium sulfate	.5 cup	138
Breakfast cereals, fortified	1 serving	130

Calcium Absorption Concerns

Vegan and nondairy diets that do not consume fish with bones should be aware of calcium absorption risks. Some vegetables and whole grains can prevent calcium absorption because they contain phytic acid and oxalate. These acids bind to the calcium and make it unusable.

- High oxalate foods: Beans, spinach, collard greens, beer, soda, chocolate, cocoa, soy (tofu, soy milk), sweet potatoes, cranberries, raspberries, wheat bran, coffee, beets, nuts, nut butters, French fries, potato chips
- High phytic acid foods: Beans, seeds, nuts, unprocessed whole grains.

The health benefits of plant-based diets are not in question. However, poorly designed vegan and vegetarian diets that do not include adequate calcium are in fact risk factors for bone-mass density issues. This is especially important for children and teens eating vegan or vegetarian diets because 90% of bone mass is created before adulthood.

Specific to RED-S and triad, when a female athlete misses menstrual cycles consistently (amenorrhea) it results in lower estrogen levels. Estrogen plays an important role in calcium absorption. Poor calcium absorption prevents healthy bone development.

A combination of a diet low in calcium-rich foods with chronic undereating and consistently missing periods creates both short-term, season-ending injury risks, but also lifelong sports career–ending concerns.

Calcium Absorption Tips

- Vitamin D helps the body absorb calcium.
- Lab tests can ensure vitamin D is at appropriate levels.
- Supplement with vitamin D if lab results indicate low levels.

VITAMIN D

Between 2017 and 2020, research studies uncovered a vitamin D deficiency pandemic. Numbers varied widely, but many adults in the United States were deficient according to various guidelines. Globally, athletes were similarly deficient. A review article found studies showing roughly 73% of athletes were vitamin D deficient.[6] There is one study showing favorable changes in biomarkers of athletes with higher (but normal) levels of vitamin D.[7]

Female Recommended Vitamin D Intake

Vitamin D (ng/mL)	Daily Intake Needs
less than 12	severely deficient
12–20	deficient
20–50	adequate
50–55	high altitude best practice
greater than 60	potentially toxic

RECOMMENDED DAILY VITAMIN D INTAKE

Vitamin D intake is not agreed upon around the world. The best practice is to have lab values drawn annually to assess vitamin D levels. There has been some difference of opinion of best vitamin D levels for sedentary people, so it is not surprising that athletes often are confused on what their levels should be. Depending on the source, either 20 or 30 ng/mL is considered the lower limit of normal. Less would be deficient and less than 12 would be severely deficient. A value of greater than 50 ng/mL is often desired in high-altitude athletes or endurance athletes, including some sources recommending up to 75 ng/mL.[8] Levels higher than 150 ng/mL are associated with vitamin D toxicity, often from overingestion.[9]

SOURCES OF VITAMIN D

There are not many foods containing vitamin D unless they have been fortified.

Foods with Vitamin D	Serving Size	IU/Serving
Salmon	3 ounces	570
Button mushroom	½ cup	366
Milk (fortified)	1 cup	120
Juice and milk alternative (fortified)	1 cup	100–144
Breakfast cereals (fortified)	1 serving	80
Egg, large	1 each	44

Vitamin D Absorption Concerns

Athletes with some conditions or genetics may have trouble absorbing key nutrients including vitamin D. These include celiac disease, irritable bowel syndrome (IBS), darker skin pigmentation, those that cover skin for SPF protection, and those who experience longer winters.

Vitamin D Absorption Tips

- Take supplements with meals that contain fat like nuts, cheese, meats, or avocados.
- Sensible skin exposure to sun.

AN ATHLETE'S STORY: Kyra

I wanted to get a Division 1 scholarship for swimming. I won the 200 and 500 freestyle at state in my sophomore year of high school. That year I made sure I didn't eat much. The skinnier I became, the faster my times were. I stopped getting my period, but I did not care. It was less to deal with each month. My junior year, I was so tired all the time. My parents took me to a doctor and I was diagnosed with an eating disorder, but my mom told the doctor it wasn't true. My mom wouldn't accept it because she had one also. She told the doctor it was a mistake, but I knew they were correct and I had no intention of fixing it.

My whole day revolved around my next meal, or skipping meals. I became skinnier and skinnier. I weighed 90 pounds and was 5 feet 6. I started feeling dizzy and lightheaded. I fainted and was diagnosed with an abnormal heart rhythm. I was put in a recovery house for eating disorders. I tried to avoid food there but they were watching us all the time. I managed to eat enough and fool them into thinking I was better and was allowed to go home. I was told I could swim again if I kept my weight on. That lasted about a month. I went back to my old ways. I felt like the only thing in my life I could control was eating. I managed to graduate from high school and was accepted to college. My parents were really afraid to let me go. In college, I kept my weight really low, but high enough that my parents would keep paying tuition. I met a guy who I really liked. We dated several months and he broke up with me saying he couldn't watch me starve myself anymore. I hit rock bottom. My grades suffered and I dropped out of school. I went back to the eating disorder program. This time I gave it a true try. It was not easy and I have had many setbacks. But I am doing a lot better and going back to school. I haven't gotten strong enough to go back to competitive swimming and I am not fast enough to make the team anymore. But I want to swim again for enjoyment at some point.

CITATIONS

1. Desbrow B, McCormack J, Burke LM, et al. Sports Dietitians Australia Position Statement: Sports Nutrition for the Adolescent Athlete. *Int J Sport Nutr Exerc Metab.* 2014; 24(5): 570–584. doi:10.1123/ijsnem.2014-0031.
2. Houltham SD, Rowlands DS. A Snapshot of Nitrogen Balance in Endurance-Trained Women. *Appl Physiol Nutr Metab.* 2014; 39(2): 219–225. doi:10.1139/apnm-2013-0182.
3. Thomas DT, Erdman KA, Burke LM. Position of the Academy of Nutrition and Dietetics, Dietitians of Canada, and the American College of Sports Medicine: Nutrition and Athletic Performance. *J Acad Nutr Diet.* 2016; 116(3): 501–528. doi: 10.1016/j.jand.2015.12.006.
4. Iron—Health Professional Fact Sheet. https://ods.od.nih.gov/factsheets/Iron-Health Professional/. Accessed June 15, 2021.
5. Rodenberg RE, Gustafson S. Iron as an Ergogenic Aid. *Curr Sports Med Rep.* 2007; 6(4): 258–264. doi:10.1097/01.csmr.0000306481.00283.f6.
6. de la Puente Yagüe M, Collado Yurrita L, Ciudad Cabañas MJ, Cuadrado Cenzual MA. Role of Vitamin D in Athletes and Their Performance: Current Concepts and New Trends. *Nutrients.* 2020; 12(2): 579. Published 2020 Feb 23. doi:10.3390/nu12020579.
7. Żebrowska A, Sadowska-Krępa E, Stanula A, et al. The Effect of Vitamin D Supplementation on Serum Total 25(OH) Levels and Biochemical Markers of Skeletal Muscles in Runners. *J Int Soc Sports Nutr.* 2020; 17(1): 18. Published 2020 Apr 9. doi:10.1186/s12970-020-00347-8.
8. Owens DJ, Allison R, Close GL. Vitamin D and the Athlete: Current Perspectives and New Challenges. *Sports Med.* 2018; 48(Suppl 1): 3–16. doi:10.1007/s40279-017-0841-9.
9. Marcinowska-Suchowierska E, Kupisz-Urbańska M, Łukaszkiewicz J, Płudowski P, Jones G. Vitamin D Toxicity—A Clinical Perspective. *Front Endocrinol (Lausanne).* 2018; 9: 550.

3 Nutrition in Training
Putting It on the Plate

Kathryn Vidlock
Rocky Vista University, Parker, CO, USA

Catherine Liggett
University of Colorado School of Medicine, Aurora, CO, USA

Elyssa Goldstein
HealthONE Family Medicine Residency, Aurora, CO, USA

CONTENTS

DOI: 10.1201/b23228-3

WORDS TO KNOW

FODMAP   Acronym for Fermentable Oligosaccharides, Disaccharides, Monosaccharides, and Polyols. These are groups that may cause GI sensitivity for athletes.

GI   Gastrointestinal; involving the digestive tract including the stomach and small and large intestines.

GLUTEN   A protein found in grains like wheat, barley, and rye.

LACTOSE   A protein found in milk and dairy products.

TRAINING PLATE MODEL   A tool used to make it easy to get the right nutrients for busy athletes.

THE TRAINING PLATE MODEL

The training plate model can be an excellent tool for athletes just starting to get into sports nutrition. The idea behind the training plate model is to modify the ratio of nutrient intake based on the intensity of exercise for the day. For example, the high-intensity training plate focuses on carbohydrate intake because more aggressive physical activity depletes glycogen stores to a greater degree. By increasing carbohydrate intake, athletes can aim to replenish these depleted energy stores, enhancing energy levels, recovery, and general health.

It is important to note that the intention of the training plate model is to alter the ratio of nutrient intake, not to restrict portion sizes. Athletes are encouraged to follow their hunger and to help themselves to a second plate if they are still hungry following their first serving. When getting a second helping, athletes should aim to still follow the ratios of the intended training plate for that day while fulfilling hunger cues.

The training plate model can be a useful tool for high school athletes due to the simplicity of its use. As athletes advance their understanding of nutrition, they may find they are able to progress past the training plate model to more individualized sports nutrition. It is important to note that the training plate model is a generalized approach to sports nutrition and certain athletes may have unique needs that require them to utilize different approaches to their nutrition. For example, athletes with certain health conditions, such as diabetes mellitus, may need to alter their carbohydrate intake in a way that differs from that prescribed by the training plate model. Certain athletes, such as endurance-based athletes, may also require increased carbohydrate intake due to significant glycogen store depletion during activity. Each athlete is different and will have unique nutritional requirements.

A limitation of the training plate model that is important to discuss is its inability to ensure, with certainty, appropriate intake of certain macro- and micronutrients. Because the training plate model urges athletes to follow their hunger cues, athletes who experience lack of appetite, have a perception of underfueling as necessary for their sport, or struggle with disordered eating/eating disorder can follow the intended ratios of the training plate model while still underfueling due to insufficient portion sizes. To illustrate this, if two athletes follow the moderate-intensity training plate but one athlete uses a 5″-diameter plate while the other uses a 10″-diameter plate, this will lead to discrepancies in nutrient intake. These discrepancies may or may not be contributory towards underfueling. Athletes looking for a more advanced sports nutrition approach are recommended to review the macronutrient section for evidence-based nutrient intake recommendations.

The training plate model utilizes three different plates as described below.

LOW-INTENSITY TRAINING PLATE

The low-intensity training plate is intended for rest days or light recovery days (e.g. stretching, walking, yoga). This plate emphasizes vegetables and fruits to increase micronutrient intake and promote recovery.

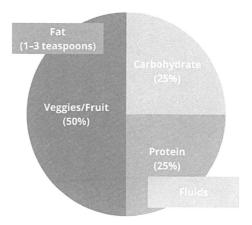

MODERATE-INTENSITY TRAINING PLATE

The moderate-intensity training plate is intended to act as a "baseline" training plate. This plate is meant to be used for the average training day (e.g. skills-based practice with a lift afterwards or base run/swim/cycle). This plate has an even ratio of carbohydrates, protein, and color (vegetables/fruit).

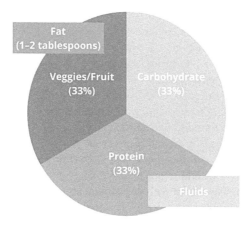

HIGH-INTENSITY TRAINING PLATE

The high-intensity training plate is intended for strenuous workouts (e.g. long runs or high-intensity interval workouts), two-a-day practices, and pre-competition/competition fueling. Because higher-intensity activity depletes glycogen stores more significantly, athletes want to increase carbohydrate intake on these days. For this reason, half of the high-intensity training plate is carbohydrates.

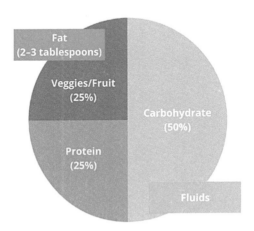

PUTTING IT INTO ACTION

Remember, almost any of these combinations will work for the plates as it depends on the ratio you use. On a low-intensity day, an athlete may just want to double up on fruit or vegetables and on a high-intensity day they may want to add more of the carbohydrate portions.

Breakfast Ideas

- Fruit salad, toast with peanut butter
- Scrambled eggs, croissant, and melon
- Avocado toast, ham, and strawberries
- Blueberry pancakes with sausage and grapes
- Rice cakes with peanut butter and clementines
- Waffles with cream cheese, strawberries, and eggs
- Omelet with cheese, peppers, broccoli, and toast
- Oatmeal with apple chunks and sausage
- Chickpea and avocado toast and raspberries
- Quinoa with milk, hard-boiled egg, and grapefruit
- On the go—Bagel with hummus and a peach
- On the go—English muffin with egg or ham and a banana
- On the go—Protein bar with orange (protein bars often have carbohydrates also)

- On the go—Bagel with peanut butter and apple
- On the go—Breakfast burrito with egg, peppers, mushrooms, and onion
- On the go—Granola bar with hard-boiled egg and a plum

Lunch Ideas

- Grilled cheese and ham sandwich with tomato soup
- Broccoli and cheese soup with bread
- Chicken breast with rice and asparagus
- Taco in a bag
- Sweet and sour chicken with squash and zucchini
- Spinach and berry smoothie with cheese and crackers
- Salami sandwich with cheese, broccoli spears, and grapes
- Pizza slice with side salad
- On the go—Pita bread with hummus, carrot slices, and melon slices
- On the go—Peanut butter sandwich with a peach
- On the go—Garden salad with roast beef sandwich
- On the go—Celery with peanut butter, apple, crackers, and cheese
- On the go—Croissant with chicken salad and grapes
- On the go—Pretzels with chunks of cheese, pear slices, chickpeas

Dinner Ideas

- Pad Thai with shrimp over rice
- Beef enchiladas with cheese, roasted tomatoes, and zucchini
- Chef salad with bread
- Roast beef with sourdough bread and roasted Brussel sprouts
- Pizza with sausage, peppers, and onions
- Pho with beef, carrots, baby corn, and onions
- Baked chicken with potatoes, broccoli, and cauliflower
- Stew with beef, potatoes, and mixed vegetables

NUTRITION ON A BUDGET

Maintaining a balanced and nutritious diet doesn't need to break the bank. The goal of this section is to discuss ways to mitigate the high price of high-protein foods, healthy grains, fruits, and vegetables. Often, athletes have tight schedules and high-caloric demands. Planning and preparing healthy meals is key to maintaining adequate nutrition on a tight budget. In addition to reviewing how to make a successful meal plan and list, we will discuss what foods to buy in bulk and other considerations for maintaining a budget-friendly diet.

MAKING A MEAL PLAN AND LIST

Eliminating food waste and avoiding the drive-thru after practice are two of many reasons athletes should plan food in anticipation of their weekly needs. Meal planning, shopping, and, in some cases, preparing food on an off day should be considered as part of a wholesome training plan. During this time, it is important for the athlete to assess what foods in their pantry and refrigerator need to be replaced and what foods are already adequately supplied. If foods have spoiled, the athlete should thoughtfully consider why.

Consider the following: Was too much purchased? Was produce not carefully evaluated before purchase, and therefore spoiled quickly? Was the food pushed to the back of the pantry/refrigerator and forgotten? These questions will help guide future food purchases.

Once supply has been assessed, the budget-conscious athlete should consider what meals they plan to eat for the week. As previously mentioned, every athlete will have different demands. It is important to consider the training plate model and portion size when shopping for food. In addition, variety in the weekly meal plan can be achieved while conserving time and money by using several of the same ingredients in different ways. For example, an athlete may purchase one large package of lean ground beef that can be used for hamburgers and spaghetti bolognese. Chicken can be used to make chicken parmesan and chicken fajitas. By carefully planning weekly meals and reusing ingredients in different ways, it is possible to maintain variety. This same approach can be applied to meal preparation, and athletes can purchase one set of ingredients to make a variety of meals for the week.

Meal planning and creating a list of necessary ingredients prior to a shopping trip not only saves money, it also saves time. By having a plan and the necessary food supply for the week, the athlete can successfully plan time to prepare food, whether that is once per week or on a nightly basis. Some may choose to plan to make leftovers, too. If this is the case, leftovers that will not be eaten within 1–2 days can be frozen in single-portion sizes to be consumed at a later date. This can be convenient for busy weeks with little time to prepare food.

WHAT TO BUY AND HOW TO BUY IT

Certain foods are best purchased in bulk while others should be bought on an as-needed basis. Every athlete should have a few nutrient-dense staples in their pantry or refrigerator at all times. In general, prepared foods are more expensive and less nutritious than homemade options. With that said, occasionally purchasing prepared foods can be helpful for athletes on a tight schedule. Here we will include lists and explanations of foods the athlete should and shouldn't purchase in bulk.

Foods to purchase in bulk:

1. *Dried beans and lentils:* These are full of protein, full of fiber, and simple to prepare! Dried beans are less expensive per serving than their canned counterparts and don't have any added sodium. Better yet, they can be used in a variety of dishes or serve as a high-protein snack. Dried beans have a minimum shelf life of 1–2 years, and there are several online retailers who sell them in bulk.
2. *Oats:* Oats are a wonderful source of much-needed carbohydrates, are versatile, and can be prepared quickly. With a shelf life of 12 months to 2 years,

it is certainly reasonable to purchase a large package of oats. Just make sure they are properly stored in an airtight container. It is also more cost effective to flavor oats with fresh fruit or brown sugar at home than to purchase individual flavored packets of oatmeal.

3. *Poultry and meat:* Purchasing any form of meat can be expensive. Watch for sales at your local grocery store, and keep an eye out for buy-one-get-one deals. Meat can be frozen and used at a later time, so it is best purchased at its lowest price point. In addition, consider purchasing a larger package of meat and freezing the rest when doing weekly grocery shopping. Freeze any that won't be used within the next 2–3 days, and plan to thaw it before your next grocery trip. This can prevent having to purchase meat on a weekly basis.

4. *Protein powder:* Many protein powders have shelf lives of at least 2 years. Athletes who use protein powder generally consume it regularly, so consider purchasing this item in bulk. Online retailers often sell protein powders in large quantities, and the athlete may even be able to get a discount on several different flavors of protein powder in one order.

5. *Greek yogurt:* Although not necessarily in bulk, it is more cost-effective to purchase large tubs of Greek yogurt rather than individual servings. The athlete may use reusable containers to pack portions and add fruits, granola, or chia seeds.

6. *Dark chocolate:* This is a great treat to stock up on. Unopened dark chocolate has a shelf life of 2 years. Once opened, it has a shelf life of one year. This same rule does not apply to other milk-containing chocolates.

7. *Pasta:* Another great source of necessary carbohydrates to fuel training, competition, and recovery. Dry pasta is best consumed within 2 years, and, as a staple in many athletes' diets, it is cost-effective to purchase in bulk.

8. *Jerky:* Although not inexpensive, jerky can be a great portable source of protein. Individual packages are usually more expensive per ounce than when purchased in bulk. At the same time it is important to remember an athlete may not be able to consume an entire large bag while it is still safe to eat. Generally, jerky is best if consumed within 3–7 days after opening. For this reason, it may be worthwhile for the athlete to consider purchasing a bulk supply of smaller packages of jerky to pay a lower price per ounce while reducing potential food waste.

9. *Nut butters:* Another common staple in athletes' pantries, nut butters can be great sources of healthy fat and protein. Online retailers sell large tubs of nut butters, and purchasing a larger portion can save money. Unopened, many of these last about 1 year in the refrigerator. Once opened, a jar of nut butter should be consumed within 2–3 months.

10. *Canned tuna:* Rather than buying small portions of canned tuna at a time, consider purchasing these in larger supply. This can save money, and many stores will have a discount if multiple packages are purchased at a time. Canned tuna is a great source of protein and will last up to 5 years in the pantry.

Foods to avoid purchasing in bulk:

1. *Fresh fruits and vegetables:* These don't have a long shelf life, so it is best not to purchase more than you can eat within a few days. If produce is routinely going to waste, consider purchasing canned fruits and vegetables. These are still nutritious options, especially if they don't contain added sugar.

   An exception to this rule is if fruits or vegetables are on sale. If this is the case, extra fruits and vegetables may be purchased and frozen immediately. When in season, certain fruits and vegetables are available at a lower cost and are at peak flavor. For example, the athlete may purchase extra blueberries (typically costly) at a lower price in June–August and freeze them for smoothies and pancakes in winter months.
2. *Eggs:* These have a shelf life of 3–5 weeks. Although eggs can be used in a variety of dishes, it is generally best not to purchase eggs in bulk if you live alone or don't eat eggs daily.
3. *Olive oil:* This may be a staple in many athletes' recipes and diets. Olive oil has a shelf life of 18–24 months once it's bottled, and only 6 months once opened. With this in mind, it is best not to purchase large or numerous bottles at a time.

OTHER CONSIDERATIONS FOR MAINTAINING A BUDGET-FRIENDLY DIET

1. Most grocery stores have an app with weekly coupons. Try choosing meals for the week based on coupons and what's already in the pantry.
2. Choose store brands; they're usually less expensive.
3. When going out to eat, refrigerate leftovers immediately. This will keep them safe to consume the following day.
4. If living with roommates or siblings, consider sharing bulk foods.
5. Sign up for a grocery loyalty/rewards program.

SPORT-SPECIFIC NEEDS

Some sports are more cardiovascular while others rely more on muscle power. How does this affect nutritional needs?

There has been some research on sports requiring both cardio and power intensity, like mid-distance running, swimming, mid-distance cycling, and rowing. Different types of training require different nutrients. Working on technical aspects requires lower carbohydrates but some protein for muscle recovery. Long aerobic training requires carbohydrates, proteins, and fats, whereas short bursts or short recovery sets require more carbohydrates and proteins.[1]

Many endurance athletes have different needs for portions of their seasons. This may include pre-/early season, mid-season, and taper portions. During the early season or preseason, depending on the sport, athletes may need more fat in addition to their carbohydrates and protein if they are working on long endurance. However, if they work on muscle gain and power in that time, they may need more protein.

During the mid-season their workouts often become more challenging, and their overall needs may be higher in carbohydrates and protein. During the taper portion of the season, there may be less need for overall calories and fat.

If an athlete is doing twice-a-day practices, it is important to remember protein—especially in the morning to help with an afternoon practice, or at a later dinner or snack to help with morning practice the next day. Nutritional needs may be high the day of competition; however, it can be hard to logistically find time to eat properly. Snacking may be of help. Athletes who have competitions that last several days need to be aware of their nutrition or they may be very fatigued by the last day.[2]

ADJUSTING FOR SPECIFIC DIETARY NEEDS

Many athletes have dietary needs that can make it challenging to follow a basic nutrition plan. But that doesn't mean that they cannot make substitutes to have good nutrition for their performances.

TRUE FOOD ALLERGIES

True food allergies are serious. An allergy is an immune response that can cause a myriad of symptoms, from mild itchiness to anaphylaxis, a life-threatening reaction. Studies estimate that around 5% of people have a true food allergy while the incidence of intolerance is higher.[3] Some children diagnosed with food allergies do outgrow them.

Food allergy symptoms can occur within a few minutes up to 2 or more hours. The most common symptoms are itchy/tingly mouth, hives, lip or facial swelling, wheezing or shortness of breath, abdominal pain, nausea, vomiting, dizziness, or lightheadedness. But sometimes anaphylaxis can occur. This is a very severe reaction consisting of narrowing of the airways, swollen throat, drop in blood pressure, rapid pulse, dizziness, or loss of consciousness. Emergent treatment with epinephrine and other supportive treatments is imperative or anaphylaxis may be fatal.

Food allergies can be caused by shellfish (shrimp, lobster, and crab), peanuts, tree nuts, fish, eggs, milk, wheat, and soy. Athletes with true food allergies need to avoid these foods and will have to pay attention to food labels and carry an EpiPen in case of accidental ingestion.

A less severe type of food allergy is oral allergy syndrome. This affects people with hay fever. Some foods have proteins that are similar to kinds of pollens, which is called cross-reactivity. Eating these foods when uncooked may trigger symptoms. Heating the foods generally denatures the proteins, so cooking them will cause less or no symptoms.

Some examples include:

- Allergy to birch pollen can cross-react with almonds, apples, apricots, carrots, cherries, hazelnuts, peaches, peanuts, pears, plums, and soybeans.
- Allergy to ragweed may cross-react with bananas, cucumbers, cantaloupe, honeydew, watermelon, and zucchini.

- Allergy to grasses may cross-react with kiwi, melons, oranges, peanuts, tomatoes, and potatoes.
- Allergy to mugwort may cross-react with apples, peppers, broccoli, cabbage, cauliflower, garlic, onions, and peaches.

Some athletes can have exercise-induced allergies. Eating suspect foods and exercising can bring on allergic symptoms, including anaphylaxis. If this occurs, athletes should eat several hours prior to exercise.

CELIAC DISEASE

Celiac disease is different than intolerance to gluten. True celiac disease is an immune-mediated response, but it is a different mechanism than a classic food allergy. It is caused by the gluten protein. Gluten is found in wheat, barley, and rye. A diagnosis is achieved by undergoing endoscopy and a biopsy of the small bowel, which shows antibodies specific for celiac disease. In people who have celiac disease the gluten protein causes damage to the surface of the intestine and decreased absorption of nutrients. Physical symptoms can be GI related, including abdominal pain, nausea, diarrhea, and bloating. Non–GI symptoms can include anemia, fatigue, vitamin deficiencies, headaches, cavities, joint pain, weakness, and osteoporosis.[4] If celiac disease goes untreated or undetected there is a higher risk of lymphoma and small bowel cancer.[5] Celiac disease is also associated with Crohn's disease, diverticulitis, and pancreatic insufficiency.[4] Athletes with celiac disease need to avoid gluten completely as even a small amount can cause issues. They will have to read food labels carefully and need to get carbohydrates from gluten-free sources.

GLUTEN SENSITIVITY

Gluten sensitivity involves the same proteins as celiac disease, but it is not the same problem. Gluten sensitivity is diagnosed by having a negative blood test for wheat allergy and celiac disease. People with gluten sensitivity may experience GI symptoms similar to those with celiac disease including abdominal pain, nausea, diarrhea, and bloating. However, gluten sensitivity doesn't lead to the longer-term problems. Athletes with gluten sensitivity should be careful to only take in small amounts of gluten that don't cause symptoms, but they do not need to avoid it like those with true celiac disease.

LACTOSE INTOLERANCE

Intolerance to lactose can decrease performance and cause severe GI distress. Symptoms often start 30 minutes to 2 hours after ingesting the lactose. Most athletes will experience pain, bloating, gas, and diarrhea, which can mimic other digestive issues. Lactose is a sugar found in milk and dairy products. Lactase is the enzyme that breaks down the sugars in milk to more digestible forms. While humans all have this enzyme at birth, the production of it tapers off at age 2–3 years. Some athletes can continue to have lactose into adulthood. But it is estimated that up to 75% of adults have a degree of lactose intolerance.[6]

Athletes who find that dairy products cause GI distress may want to avoid dairy. They may also be able to concentrate on foods with less lactose like yogurt. There are lactose-free milks and lactose supplements available to help also. It is wise to try these products on a regular training day rather than changing nutrition on a competition day. Athletes should also read product labels as milk and dairy products are often found in processed foods. Athletes may need to increase the amount of green leafy vegetables they consume to ensure they get enough calcium, or consider a calcium supplement.

FODMAP

Many athletes experience GI symptoms such as nausea, bloating, diarrhea, and constipation. There is more and more evidence pointing to certain foods causing intolerances. The FODMAP diet may be helpful to athletes with specific intolerances.

FODMAP is the acronym for Fermentable Oligosaccharides, Disaccharides, Monosaccharides, and Polyols. Oligosaccharides are fructans and galactans, and include wheat barley, rye, and lentils. The disaccharide is lactose including milk, yogurt, and dairy. The monosaccharide is fructose found in excess of glucose, such as mangoes, apples, and asparagus. Polyols are sorbitol, mannitol, xylitol, and maltitol or sugar alcohols, and are often in diet foods like sugar-free candy or gum.

A low FODMAP can be challenging to follow as it is not always obvious which foods have the substances. Using a tool such as the Monash University app can be helpful. Avoiding high-fiber foods the day of the competition or the night before may be helpful. Avoiding sugar-free foods and beans the day of competition may help also. The biggest aid is in knowing which of the categories is the issue. So, starting with avoiding all the groups and slowly introducing each back may provide insight into the substance that causes symptoms. Because it can be so complicated, athletes may want to work with a dietitian.

VEGAN OR VEGETARIAN

Athletes may use a vegan or some form of vegetarian diet. This is not impossible to do as an athlete, but it does take considerable attention to getting proteins and nutrients.[7]

There are many different classifications of vegetarian diets:

- *Vegans* avoid all animal products and are the strictest.
- *Lacto-ovo vegetarians* exclude anything with flesh but eat dairy and eggs.
- *Lacto-vegetarians* exclude flesh and eggs but will eat dairy.
- *Ovo-vegetarians* exclude flesh and dairy but eat eggs.
- *Pesco-vegetarians* exclude flesh but will eat fish.
- *Fruitarians* exclude animal products and primarily eat fruit, nuts, seeds, and some vegetables.

- *Flexitarians* try to minimize their consumption of animals but occasionally eat fish, eggs, and dairy.
- *Pollo-vegetarians* avoid meat from cows and pigs but eat poultry.
- *Pollo-pesco-vegetarians* avoid meat from cows and pigs but eat poultry and fish.

Poorly constructed diets may lead to a lack of energy, poor bone density, and deficiencies in vitamin B12, riboflavin, vitamin D, calcium, iron, and zinc. In addition, vegans and vegetarians tend to have more fiber in their diets. While this can be very healthy, it can promote a feeling of fullness earlier, causing an athlete to underfuel. Vegans especially tend to take in less protein, and the protein they consume tends to have less essential amino acids. Paying attention to how grains, legumes, nuts, and seeds are consumed can help with this issue. Athletes following a stricter type of vegetarian diet may want to consult with a sports dietitian.[7]

DIABETIC DIET

There is no reason that an athlete with controlled diabetes cannot participate in most sports. They will have to be diligent about following their blood glucose levels. Many diabetic athletes who are participating in their sport for the first time will find their caloric needs are higher and their insulin needs may change as well. Any diabetic participating in sports needs to develop a plan through their physician and dietitian.

AN ATHLETE'S STORY: Elise

I grew up on a farm in the Midwest with three older brothers. We did a lot of work and I was strong. My brothers teased me for being a girl and called me wimpy, so I always wanted to be stronger. They all played baseball and football. My parents signed me up for softball when I was in first grade. I was not very coordinated, but I was strong. Once I learned how to watch the ball, I hit home runs all the time. My dad worked with me on coordination, and I eventually started pitching. I made traveling teams easily and continued to be a strong batter.

In high school, we started strength training and my shoulders got even bigger. I felt I was heavy, but my parents told me I was a solid farm kid. Our meals had meat and gravy often and if there was salad, it was on the side. I didn't count calories, or diet. I did really well in softball and got a scholarship to college.

In college, there were other girls as big as me on the softball team. But, off the field, I felt like a large farm kid still. Our dining hall had more vegetables and salads and I tried new options. My roommate was a vegetarian studying to be a dietitian. She was really surprised by the way my family ate, because she grew up with a single mom who ate salads all the time. She taught me some healthier options. I thought this would help me to lose weight, but I only lost a few pounds.

The Exercise Science Department offered underwater weighing to determine body fat percentage. I wasn't going to do it because I felt I would be really high. But my roommate told me it would be confidential. So, I agreed. In the waiting area there were charts of percentages that were low, athletic, normal, and obese. I figured I would be obese. I did the weighing, which was different than I thought. I had to sit on a chair hanging from a diving board and then it went underwater and I had to let all my breath out. Two days later, I returned for the results. I was shocked to learn I fit into the athletic range. The grad student was not surprised because I was an athlete. She explained to me that BMI was not a good calculation for muscular females and I should ignore it. She encouraged me to keep strength training and that I could recheck every year if I wanted. I felt so relieved and so incredibly happy. This one event changed my whole perspective about myself. My confidence grew and I no longer avoided mirrors. I felt pride in my muscles.

I graduated and became an athletic trainer for a rural high school. I like to talk to the girls who look like me and encourage them to remain healthy and not fall into the trap of low self-esteem because they are muscular. I wish I had the confidence in high school that I have now. I missed out on events because I worried about my appearance. I am glad girls will be taking these classes because the problem is larger than most parents think.

CITATIONS

1. Stellingwerff T, Maughan RJ, Burke LM. Nutrition for Power Sports: Middle-Distance Running, Track Cycling, Rowing, Canoeing/Kayaking, and Swimming. *J Sports Sci.* 2011; 29(Suppl 1): S79–S89. doi:10.1080/02640414.2011.589469.
2. Jeukendrup AE. Periodized Nutrition for Athletes. *Sports Med.* 2017; 47(Suppl 1): 51–63. doi:10.1007/s40279-017-0694-2.
3. Loh W, Tang MLK. The Epidemiology of Food Allergy in the Global Context. *Int J Environ Res Public Health.* 2018; 15(9): 2043. Published 2018 Sep 18. doi:10.3390/ijerph15092043.
4. Caio G, Volta U, Sapone A, et al. Celiac Disease: A Comprehensive Current Review. *BMC Med.* 2019; 17(1): 142. Published 2019 Jul 23. doi:10.1186/s12916-019-1380-z.
5. Marafini I, Monteleone G, Stolfi C. Association between Celiac Disease and Cancer. *Int J Mol Sci.* 2020; 21(11): 4155. Published 2020 Jun 10. doi:10.3390/ijms21114155.
6. Silanikove N, Leitner G, Merin U. The Interrelationships between Lactose Intolerance and the Modern Dairy Industry: Global Perspectives in Evolutional and Historical Backgrounds. *Nutrients.* 2015; 7(9): 7312–7331. Published 2015 Aug 31. doi:10.3390/nu7095340.
7. Rogerson D. Vegan Diets: Practical Advice for Athletes and Exercisers. *J Int Soc Sports Nutr.* 2017; 14: 36. Published 2017 Sep 13. doi:10.1186/s12970-017-0192-9.

4 Advanced Nutrition

Andrew Dole

University of Waikato, Hamilton, New Zealand

Kathryn Vidlock

Rocky Vista University, Parker, CO, USA

CONTENTS

WORDS TO KNOW

FAD DIETS   Popular diets that promise weight loss or other benefits without real science to back it up.

pH BALANCE   Rating scale used to describe how acidic or basic a solution is.

SUPPLEMENTS

Supplements discussed in this chapter are all vitamins, minerals, and other over-the-counter supplements commonly used by athletes. A discussion of performance-enhancing substances is covered in Chapter 5 about nutrition going wrong.

DOI: 10.1201/b23228-4

Athletes commonly take extra vitamins or supplements to help with everyday health, attempting to prevent deficiencies, or increase performance. A survey showed that 45.2% of athletes take supplements more than two days a week and those most commonly used were vitamins and minerals at 25.5% and proteins and amino acids at 24.6%.[1]

There can be regulatory issues for athletes. It is commonly thought that over-the-counter supplements are all safe to use and allowed by athletic organizations but this can vary. For example, the sleeping aid melatonin is actually regulated by prescription in some countries, while in the United States, it is not a problem to use without a prescription.[2] Let's discuss some of the commonly used supplements.

Iron is a commonly used supplement for female athletes. Iron needs in menstruating athletes are elevated and discussed previously. There are several stages of iron deficiency, and it is reported that 24–47% of women experience iron deficiency without anemia.[3] A lack of iron can lead to a lowering of metabolism and decreased energy availability and contributes to suppression in bone health.[4] However, athletes who are not iron deficient and take supplements can cause health issues including iron toxicity. Iron levels, including ferritin, a marker of iron stores, should be measured prior to taking iron supplements and a physician should be consulted when using iron supplements.

Calcium is another commonly used supplement. Although calcium levels can be measured in the blood, it is not an accurate measurement of overall calcium status. Calcium needs may be up to 1500 mg a day in athletes who are underfueling or have menstrual irregularities. Calcium supplementation needs to be broken up and taken 2–3 times daily as our bodies generally do not absorb more than 500 mg to 600 mg at a time.[5] An excess of calcium may cause buildup in the blood vessels, so it is not advised to take more than recommended. Any athlete taking more than 1200 mg a day should consult their physician.

Vitamin D is a supplement that helps athletes to absorb calcium as well as aiding in other body systems. Vitamin D has received a lot of media attention as many people are deficient when their blood levels are measured. There is no true consensus of how much supplementation is healthy. Up to 1000 IU–2000 IU may be recommended, and in cases of deficiency, 50,000 IU a week may be prescribed. Again, consulting with a physician is recommended in cases of deficiency.[6] There is some evidence that jump height and muscle power is correlated with vitamin D levels.[7]

Zinc is a supplement commonly thought to help tissue healing and aid in healing cold-like symptoms. However, too much zinc can cause a decrease in the immune response. There is no agreement on taking zinc supplementation.[8]

Vitamins B and C are water-soluble vitamins. This means that if an athlete takes too much it will simply be excreted in their urine. There is some support for taking vitamin C in the presence of cold symptoms.[6]

Glutamine is an amino acid that may aid in the immune system and it is known that there are less circulating levels of glutamine after hard workouts. Because of that, there is a belief that supplementation will aid in recovery. But there is no agreement on how much to take and little evidence to show that it does aid recovery.[6]

Gelatin and collagen are generally thought to be safe and there is a belief that they aid in injuries to tendon and connective tissue, but more studies need to be done to provide definitive evidence.[9]

FAD DIETS

THE DANGER OF FAD DIETS

There are new fad diets each year. Each one raves about the special benefits it provides, especially for weight loss, fat burning, or toning specific parts of the body. Unfortunately, these outcomes are rarely true and are never based on science fact. Fad diets rely on hidden calorie restriction, avoidance of food groups, or the myths of superfoods. This is where they become risky for everyone but especially dangerous for the young athlete.

TOP WORST FAD DIETS

Paleo

Food choices are limited to what our caveman ancestors would have eaten. This omits grains, beans, and dairy. At the Paleo diet's extreme, it does not allow for processed or packaged foods at all.

At first, this sounds pretty good. It focuses on meats (protein), fruits, vegetables, nuts, and seeds. All those foods would make for a nutritious, well-rounded meal for the average person. However, athletes need carbohydrates to fuel their sport and young athletes need calories to fuel their growth. Avoiding all grains removes easily accessible, affordable, and nutritious sources of both calories and carbohydrates. Dairy, which often provides an affordable source of lean protein, calcium, and vitamin D, is also excluded from the Paleo diet. However, with the increase in animal meat providing amino acid–rich proteins with vitamin D the absence of dairy becomes less of a nutrition concern, but it does hurt the pocketbook for the family as well as affect convenience for the student athlete.

Pros
   Promotes eating lots of nuts, seeds, vegetables, and meats/fish that provide rich sources of protein, iron, and omega-3 fats.

Cons
   Omits grains—an important source of fiber, vitamins, minerals, and carbohydrates. Beans and legumes are not allowed, minimizing high-fiber plant-protein foods. Dairy is avoided, taking away a convenient source of lean protein and nutrients. This diet is often abused and becomes unbalanced when meat is the focus and not balanced with lots of fruits, vegetables, and other plants.

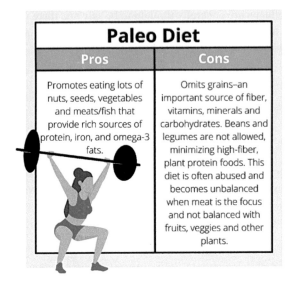

Paleo Diet	
Pros	Cons
Promotes eating lots of nuts, seeds, vegetables and meats/fish that provide rich sources of protein, iron, and omega-3 fats.	Omits grains–an important source of fiber, vitamins, minerals and carbohydrates. Beans and legumes are not allowed, minimizing high-fiber, plant protein foods. This diet is often abused and becomes unbalanced when meat is the focus and not balanced with fruits, veggies and other plants.

Ketogenic (Keto)

Eating incredibly low amounts of carbohydrates every day will put the body into nutritional ketosis. A typical ketogenic diet requires 25–75 g of carbohydrates per day to put the body into ketosis. Nutritional ketosis favors fat as the primary energy source for the body and allows the brain to use ketones instead of glucose for fuel. This ability to use both ketones or glucose is a metabolic advantage with obvious uses in times of starvation or food scarcity when abundant food sources are not available.

A ketogenic diet has many therapeutic uses and should be seen as a medical solution and an eating lifestyle for the average person. Epilepsy, cancer, obesity, and metabolic diseases like type 2 diabetes are examples of ketogenic diet uses.

However, a ketogenic diet has been proven to decrease performance in most every sport except for some ultra-distance events. Keto is not the same as fat adaptation and reduces an athlete's ability to reach high-intensity efforts. A good example would be an athlete in competition with five gears and they need all five gears to compete, but they are stuck in fourth gear all the time. You can see how that would be a problem in training or competition.

Additionally, a ketogenic diet does not allow for high-quality, nutrient-dense foods. To stay in ketosis and eat the required carbohydrates, most all grains, fruits, vegetables and even proteins must be limited severely.

Lastly, female athletes are genetically better at using fat for fuel and do not use carbohydrates optimally at high-intensity efforts. In sports that require frequent high-intensity bursts, a ketogenic diet will only further reduce their ability to reach those high-intensity needs by making their ability to access carbohydrates worse. What about endurance sports? Up to the marathon, female athletes are competing at incredibly high intensities and are still reliant on carbohydrates for fuel. Some ultra-events may potentially favor a ketogenic diet, but it is unlikely we will see mainstream youth ultra-events.

Pros
- For an athlete, there are currently no performance or health benefits.

Cons
- Severely restricts fruits, vegetables, and grains.
- Limits phytochemical intake.
- Very low fiber intake leads to chronic constipation.
- Negatively alters gut bacteria, which may affect the immune system, mental health, and digestion.
- May deprive young adults of necessary nutrients to mature properly.
- If improperly done can lead to increased cardiovascular risks from high-saturated fat intakes.
- Requires daily supplementation of many vitamins and minerals as well as sodium.

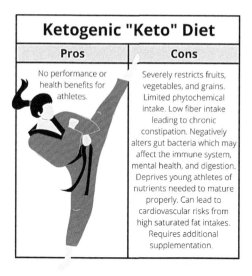

Ketogenic "Keto" Diet

Pros	Cons
No performance or health benefits for athletes.	Severely restricts fruits, vegetables, and grains. Limited phytochemical intake. Low fiber intake leading to chronic constipation. Negatively alters gut bacteria which may affect the immune system, mental health, and digestion. Deprives young athletes of nutrients needed to mature properly. Can lead to cardiovascular risks from high saturated fat intakes. Requires additional supplementation.

Intermittant Fasting

Intermittent fasting (IF), also known as time-restricted eating, has many different versions. The most popular form is to restrict when a person can eat to a set window of time. For example, 16–8 fasting would be 16 hours of food restriction that is followed by 8 hours when food can be eaten, as much and as often as they like. The perceived benefits of this are weight loss, improved blood sugar, and improved insulin sensitivity—none of which are issues young athletes should be concerned with. Furthermore, new research has not successfully shown that fasting provides any of these benefits, and that weight loss is the side effect of eating fewer calories over the whole day. However, weight and appearance are common goals for young athletes and intermittent fasting may be something they turn to.

Unfortunately, it is hard enough to get young athletes to eat all the calories and nutrients they need in a whole day. Limiting the hours of when they can eat will only make this worse and lead to chronic undereating.

Another problem is that weekly training sessions in youth sports are never black and white. There are rarely easy days or hard days and almost always have a mixture of low-intensity and high-intensity work with quite a bit of skill-based practice. These types of activities require sufficient carbohydrates and energy from meals to get the most out of them.

Lastly, when you add in the limitations of eating quality food during a school day with time-restricted eating, intermittent fasting becomes a harmful diet practice.

Pros
- For the young athlete there are no performance or health benefits from inter-mittent fasting.

Cons
- Restricts time an athlete can eat.
- Teaches a young athlete to dismiss their natural hunger signals.
- Usually results in too few calories and nutrients being consumed every day.

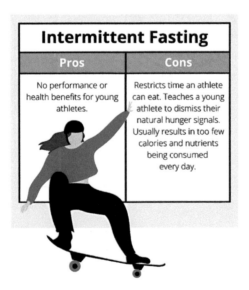

Intermittent Fasting	
Pros	**Cons**
No performance or health benefits for young athletes.	Restricts time an athlete can eat. Teaches a young athlete to dismiss their natural hunger signals. Usually results in too few calories and nutrients being consumed every day.

Alkaline Diets

The idea behind this diet is that certain foods are acidic or alkaline (acid or base), and by avoiding acid-forming foods, it is possible to change the pH balance (acidity) of our blood.

The diet recommends avoiding meats, most grains, some nuts, dairy, sugar, and processed foods because they are acid forming.

Foods like fruits, vegetable, seeds, and some nuts are considered alkaline and good for you.

This is a highly restrictive diet that omits many nutritious food groups to achieve an impossible goal— changing blood pH balance. The pH of the blood (7.35–7.4) is important for normal cell function and body processes to occur. Needless to say, the body tightly regulates blood pH with the help of the lungs, kidneys, and buffer compounds in the cells.

Also, regardless of the types of foods we eat, they are digested with a powerful acid in the stomach. A plate full of alkaline foods would be made more acidic through the digestion process. How does the body prevent food leaving the stomach from eating through the intestines? The acidic blob of chewed-up food is neutralized with bile as it enters the small intestine for absorption to the bloodstream.

As you can imagine, there is no science to support an alkaline diet for blood pH. However, eating lots of fruits and vegetables is beneficial when done without the highly restrictive nature of this diet.

Pros
- Eating lots of fruits and vegetables will always be beneficial for health.

Cons
- Incredibly restrictive.
- Omits accessible and affordable protein sources.
- Restricts valuable carbohydrate and fiber sources.
- No science to support it.

Blood Type Diets

The blood type diet claims to improve health and reduce the risk of diseases like cancer and cardiovascular disease. Different food types are suggested depending on which of the four blood types (A, B, AB, O) the person has.

- *Type A* has an increased risk of cardiovascular disease and is directed to eat a vegetarian diet.
- *Type B* should eat plants and meats but should avoid chicken or pork.
- *Type AB* can eat a wide variety of foods but is advised to avoid certain beans, corn, chicken, and beef.
- *Type O* should eat lean proteins and certain fruits and vegetables while limiting dairy, grains, and beans.

Despite its popularity and 20-year lifespan this diet has no evidence to support it. In fact, several studies were unable to find any association with blood type and diet interventions.

With no evidence to prove any of the health claims this diet makes, it also has no therapeutic or diagnostic uses, making it one of the worst fad diets.

Pros

There are no benefits to this diet.

Cons

Certain blood types must restrict foods and food groups.

Whole 30

The Whole 30 diet is a strict-elimination diet meant for short-term use—30 days. The diet claims to stop sugar cravings, reduce inflammation, improve immune system function, repair the gut, and more.

By design, an elimination diet removes foods from the diet. Sometimes this is done as a diagnostic to uncover allergies, sensitivities, or intolerances. Once identified, foods are added back into the diet. Unfortunately, many people have decided to take this 30-day diet and turn it into everyday forever eating.

Whole 30 has a very strict allowed and avoided list of foods. Whole 30 does promote eating lots of fruits, vegetables, and lean proteins, which is the cornerstone to a performance diet. Beyond that, there some glaring issues with this diet.

First, there are quite a few inconsistencies when it comes to why some foods are allowed and others are omitted. For example, an allowed seed may have higher levels of the nutrient they are trying to avoid than a food on the avoid list.

Second, many of the foods omitted such as dairy, legumes, and whole grains have science to suggest they help decrease inflammation, not cause it.

Third, it starts a negative and unhelpful relationship with foods by promoting a Good Food vs. Bad Food mentality.

Pros
- Reduces the amount of processed foods in the diet.
- Promotes more whole foods.

Cons
- Mentality of "30 days and it's over".
- Good Food vs. Bad Food design.
- Eliminates food groups that help fight inflammation.
- Restricts entire foods groups.
- Inconsistencies in the foods allowed and avoided.

Whole 30 Diet	
Pros	**Cons**
Reduces amount of processed food in the diet. Promotes more whole foods.	30 days of health is not equivalent to life-long health. Good food vs. bad food design negative for general health. Eliminates food groups that help fight inflammation. Restricts entire food groups. Inconsistencies in foods allowed and avoided.

Cleanses and Detoxes

Detox and cleanse diets claim to remove toxic buildup of waste and chemicals in the body. They are also used to jump-start fat loss. In reality they are short-term, highly restrictive, fasting diets that have never been support by science. In fact, they are absolutely the worst diet any human, especially an athlete, could ever use. These diets only harm, promote unhealthy eating habits, and most importantly are completely unnecessary.

The human body detoxifies itself every day. The liver, kidneys, lungs, sweat, lymph system, feces, and urine all work together to process and eliminate waste in the body. This is well-researched human physiology. On the other hand, not one research study has ever shown a detox or cleanse diet to remove toxins from the body.

Additionally, these crash-style diets drastically reduce calories, promote excess hydration, limit intake to juice, herbs, or spices and are unable to supply the body with adequate nutrition to fuel daily life, repair, and recovery. The detox itself can be more stressful on the body than the toxins they claim to remove.

Athletes thinking about using detox or cleanse diets risk stressing the human body and compromising performance potential.

Pros

- It is tough to place any positives in this column. To be fair, drinking more water, avoiding sugar, omitting processed foods, and eating lots of fruits or vegetables are all healthful habits, but following a highly restrictive detox/ cleanse diet is not necessary to do these things. These habits should be part of a daily eating routine that provides adequate calories, protein, and nutrients to promote recovery, repair, and performance gains.

Cons
- Stressful both mentally and physically.
- Energy restrictive.
- Nutrient deficient.
- Doesn't actually do anything.
- No science to support claims.

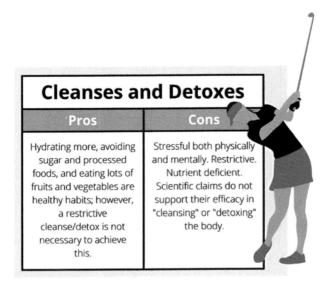

Cleanses and Detoxes	
Pros	**Cons**
Hydrating more, avoiding sugar and processed foods, and eating lots of fruits and vegetables are healthy habits; however, a restrictive cleanse/detox is not necessary to achieve this.	Stressful both physically and mentally. Restrictive. Nutrient deficient. Scientific claims do not support their efficacy in "cleansing" or "detoxing" the body.

NUTRITION DURING INJURIES

Sadly, injuries happen in athletics. There is mixed data on how nutrition may or may not help with rehabilitation. When athletes are sedentary, muscle mass decreases as well as strength and function. Many times, athletes think they should cut back the calories while recovering, but this is a mistake. An athlete's body has a higher metabolic rate while recovering from an injury and will need nutrients. If an athlete needs to use crutches, their energy need is even higher. Fueling less during this time may mean nutrients are not present for timely healing. Physicians often recommend that athletes do not lose weight and even gain a few pounds during healing.

Protein—especially whey protein—is known to help with muscle mass retention after injuries. The amino acids leucine and lysine help to regulate protein and contribute to retention of muscle mass. Having adequate carbohydrates may help with protein synthesis, but again data is mixed.[10] There is a lot to be learned about micronutrients as well. While there have been studies showing omega-3 fatty acids may be anti–inflammatory, this was not reproduced in other studies.[11] Vitamin A is helpful in healing, vitamin C aids in collagen production, and vitamin D is used in bone formation—although data is unclear if it is useful to supplement unless there is a deficiency.[12] Most professionals do not recommend overconsumption of vitamins during this time, but if you are concerned about an insufficiency, consult a physician. Hydration is important while healing and adequate fluids help with metabolism during healing.

So, how does this look for a regular meal? It may help to think about the training plates again. During healing, using a training plate that is roughly 1/3 protein, 1/3 carbohydrates, and 1/3 veggies and fruits is a good solution—this is the moderate-intensity training plate. If an athlete is less hungry, maintain the protein and vegetables and lighten the carbohydrates—this is the light-intensity training plate.

SLEEP

Sleep is important for overall function, including academic and athletic performance. High school athletes often are not sleeping enough. Teenagers 14–18 years old need between 7–10 hours of sleep each night; however, the majority of teens get about 7.5–8.5 hours of sleep each night.[13] Napping in this age group can suggest sleep deficiency. Combining academics, sports, jobs, and home responsibilities can be very difficult. Many high school athletes simply sacrifice sleep for other activities.[14]

A loss of sleep often happens during two different points in the season. First, it may happen during normal training. Athletes may be busy with homework, work, or simply staying up too late. The other time is the night before competition. Athletes may feel anxious and solving sleep problems the night before is difficult, thus maintaining an adequate sleep amount the majority of the season is key.

Athletic performance is affected by a lack of sleep. Performance is affected more with additional sleep loss, therefore one night of poor sleep may not have a big effect, but many nights of partial sleep deprivation may have a large effect. There are a few studies showing decreased function in fast reaction times and to a lesser amount, gross motor function (strength, power, and endurance).[15,16] One study has shown that athletes who get more sleep may have faster reaction times, increased energy, and more accuracy in free-throws.[17]

HOW DO SLEEP AND NUTRITION INTERACT?

Adequate sleep allows normal hormonal function and metabolism. Functions like protein production, usage of amino acids and breakdown of carbohydrates are all optimized when sleep is adequate. Appetite can change with a lack of sleep. A lack of sleep can also affect the release of melatonin—a hormone involved in regulation of sleep. Melatonin is normally released at night prior to sleep; however, in sleep-deprived individuals, release of melatonin may shift, contributing to daytime fatigue.

NAPS

Can an athlete make up for poor sleep by napping? There are few studies, but one did show that sprinting times and fatigue were improved after lunchtime naps when there had been partial sleep deprivation.[18] It is possible that athletes may benefit from napping, especially if they have early morning or late-night practice or competitions. That may be unrealistic at times for busy student athletes.

Tips to improve sleep:

- Don't nap too close to bedtime (within a few hours).
- Keep your room cold and dark.
- Keep a consistent schedule.
- Consume caffeine early in the day.

AN ATHLETE'S STORY: Bri

I loved to tumble and started gymnastics very young. I spent my recess time doing flips and handsprings with other girls. As I started getting more and more serious about gymnastics, I needed to change gyms. I was accepted into the top gym in our town. I was really proud of myself. The coaches talked about the commitment and sacrifice it would take to be really good. I was willing to do anything. I was dieting constantly by the age of 11. I limited myself to 700–800 calories a day. I counted constantly. It worked. I was praised by my coaches for remaining thin and I was winning and improving.

My parents did not like my eating habits. They constantly tried to feed me hamburgers, pizza, and other foods they thought would tempt me. But I refused. My body had to be perfect to compete. As I went through my teen years, I remained petite and stick thin. I didn't get my period. I didn't develop breasts. That was fine with me but not with my parents.

By the time I was 17, I still had not gone through puberty. I was still counting calories. I was thin and looked like an elite gymnast. But my body was done. I was fainting during practices. I was weak and tired and had trouble learning new skills. I didn't make the team I had set my goal on.

My mom forced me to go to the doctor. She said that either I went or she would stop paying for gymnastics. My mom told her about my eating habits and the lack of cycles. She also told her she didn't like the attitude of the team and that some of the other parents seemed to be encouraging the lack of food and overcommitment from their kids so it seemed normal. That was the first time I had heard my mom comment on the coaching. I thought my mom was misunderstanding. I tried to interject and explain that she didn't understand the sacrifice it took. I reiterated some of the things my coaches had said. But neither my mom or the doctor was willing to agree with me.

I had to be on a plan to gain some weight and get my cycles. I was not on board with this but it was the only way my mom would pay for gymnastics. So, I did the bare minimum required. My coaches were concerned with my weight gain. They talked to my mom about it and it did not go over well. My parents took me out of that gym and put me back into my previous gym. I was devastated.

It took me many years to realize how unhealthy this gym was for me. I feel I was brainwashed in a way. So were the other girls. This same gym produced many elite level gymnasts. Most of them have disordered eating and other issues. I am glad to see the gym is under pressure now to encourage healthy eating but I suspect much of it is all for their image and no real substance is behind it. More parents need to be educated to stand up for the health of their daughters. Athletes need to stand up for themselves. Until that happens, this will not change.

CITATIONS

1. Barrack MT, Muster M, Nguyen J, Rafferty A, Lisagor T. An Investigation of Habitual Dietary Supplement Use among 557 NCAA Division I Athletes. *J Am Coll Nutr.* 2020; 39(7):619–627. doi:10.1080/07315724.2020.1713247.
2. Dwyer JT, Coates PM, Smith MJ. Dietary Supplements: Regulatory Challenges and Research Resources. *Nutrients.* 2018; 10(1):41. Published 2018 Jan 4. doi:10.3390/nu10010041.
3. Rowland T. Iron Deficiency in Athletes: An Update. *Am J Lifestyle Med.* 2012; 6(4): 319–327. doi:10.1177/1559827611431541.
4. Petkus DL, Murray-Kolb LE, De Souza MJ. The Unexplored Crossroads of the Female Athlete Triad and Iron Deficiency: A Narrative Review. *Sports Med.* 2017; 47: 1721–1737. doi:10.1007/s40279-017-0706-2.
5. Thomas DT, Erdman KA, Burke LM. American College of Sports Medicine Joint Position Statement. Nutrition and Athletic Performance. *Med Sci Sports Exerc* 2016; 48: 543–568. 10.1249/MSS.0000000000000852.
6. Maughan RJ, Burke LM, Dvorak J, et al. IOC Consensus Statement: Dietary Supplements and the High-Performance Athlete. *Br J Sports Med.* 2018; 52(7):439–455. doi:10.1136/bjsports-2018-099027.
7. Ogan D, Pritchett K. Vitamin D and the Athlete: Risks, Recommendations, and Benefits. *Nutrients.* 2013; 5(6): 1856–1868. Published 2013 May 28. doi:10.3390/nu5061856.
8. Singh M, Das RR. Zinc for the Common Cold. *Cochrane Database Syst Rev* 2013; 6: CD001364.
9. Shaw G, Lee-Barthel A, Ross ML, et al. Vitamin C-Enriched Gelatin Supplementation before Intermittent Activity Augments Collagen Synthesis. *Am J Clin Nutr* 2017; 105: 136–43.10.3945/ajcn.116.138594.
10. Papadopoulou SK. Rehabilitation Nutrition for Injury Recovery of Athletes: The Role of Macronutrient Intake. *Nutrients.* 2020; 12(8): 2449. Published 2020 Aug 14. doi:10.3390/nu12082449.
11. Quintero KJ, de Sá Resende A, Leite GSF, Lancha Junior AH. An Overview of Nutritional Strategies for Recovery Process in Sports-Related Muscle Injuries. *Nutrire.* 2018; 43: 27. doi:10.1186/s41110-018-0084-z.
12. Papadopoulou SK, Mantzorou M, Kondyli-Sarika F, et al. The Key Role of Nutritional Elements on Sport Rehabilitation and the Effects of Nutrients Intake. *Sports (Basel).* 2022; 10(6): 84. Published 2022 May 26. doi:10.3390/sports10060084.
13. Reilly T, Deykin T. Effects of Partial Sleep Loss on Subjective States, Psychomotor and Physical Performance Tests. *J. Hum. Move. Stud.* 1983; 9: 157–170.
14. Carter HL. Common Sleep Disorders in Children. *Am Fam Physician.* 2014 Mar 1; 89(5): 368–377.
15. Reilly T, Hales A. Effects of Partial Sleep Deprivation on Performance Measures in Females. In: ED McGraw (Ed.), *Contemporary Ergonomics.* London: Taylor & Francis, 1988, pp. 509–513.
16. Reilly T, Piercy M.. The Effect of Partial Sleep Deprivation on Weight-Lifting Performance. *Ergonomics.* 1994; 37: 107–15.
17. Mah CD, Mah KE, Kezirian EJ, Dement WC. The Effects of Sleep Extension on the Athletic Performance of Collegiate Basketball Players. *Sleep.* 2011; 34: 943–950.
18. PostolacheTT, D.A. Oren. Circadian Phase Shifting, Alerting, and Antidepressant Effects of Bright Light Treatment. *Clin. Sports Med.* 2005; 24: 381–413.

5 When Nutrition Goes Wrong

Kathryn Vidlock

Rocky Vista University, Parker, CO, USA

Catherine Liggett

University of Colorado School of Medicine, Aurora, CO, USA

CONTENTS

WORDS TO KNOW

PERFORMING-ENHANCING DRUG (PED)   Any substance that is used to improve sports performance. Some of these substances are banned by various organizations.

DOI: 10.1201/b23228-5

WHAT CAN GO WRONG WITH NUTRITION?

Technically, many things can go wrong with nutrition, including the wrong amounts of nutrients or calories, as discussed previously. Use of performance-enhancing drugs is a bigger issue than many people realize. The other area that can be a problem is eating disorders. Both will be discussed here.

WHAT ARE PERFORMANCE-ENHANCING DRUGS?

Technically, performing-enhancing drugs (PEDs) are any substances that can aid in improving an athlete's performance. Some PEDs are commonly used, such as caffeine. Caffeine has been shown in studies to increase focus and alertness. Many athletes use it without any negative consequences. But most of the time the term PED is used to mean a banned substance.

WHAT PED SUBSTANCES ARE BANNED?

There are large lists of banned substances. Different athletic organizations have slightly different lists. So, athletes should be aware of the list for whichever organization they compete within. Some are completely banned and others may need a therapeutic exemption to be used (for example, an athlete with ADHD may need a therapeutic exemption to use Adderall while competing in the NCAA). Some of the more common substances used with negative consequences by teens include:

Anabolic Steroids—These are used to increase muscle mass and strength. They stimulate the appetite and help athletes to gain weight. They can be thought of as similar in structure and action to the hormone testosterone. Athletes may use these in intermittent bursts or cycle through periods of using them. No specific timing of their use is proven to be more effective. Most often they are used in sports where strength is an advantage, such as weightlifting, football, rugby, etc. Athletes taking steroids usually do not have the same type of "high" that other drugs may bring. These are banned across all athletic organizations. Examples include nandrolone, oxandrolone, oxymetholone, stanozolol, and trenbolone acetate.

Anabolic Steroid Precursors—These are substances that are converted into anabolic steroids by our bodies. Examples include androstenedione (andro) and dehydroepiandrosterone (DHEA). DHEA is of special note as it is available without a prescription and is a precursor to both testosterone and estrogen. The effects of these supplements are similar to the effects of steroids.

Human Growth Hormone—This is used to build muscle mass and strength. It is also known as hGH. It can be used in combination with anabolic steroids or with erythropoietin (EPO) to increase power and strength. It is very hard to detect as a doping agent as this hormone is normally found in humans.

Amphetamines and Stimulants—These are used to increase focus and endurance. Examples include Ritalin and Adderall. Many students use stimulants to treat ADHD and can get therapeutic exemptions if needed for their sport. Most high school leagues do not require this for high school athletes, but other athletic organizations may require it.

Creatine—This is used to increase muscle mass and help with high-intensity sports. It is available over the counter. It can be found in energy supplements and drinks and is often not advertised on the label. It is not banned in most athletic organizations but does have risks.

HOW DO TEENS GET THESE SUBSTANCES?

Unfortunately, these substances are widely available. Teens are often able to get these through other students or by asking at gyms. A cycle of steroids may last about 10 weeks and cost as little as $60–$80.[1]

ARE PEDs HARMFUL?

PEDs have many harmful effects.

Steroids and steroid precursors
- Loss of normal growth in height
- High blood pressure
- High cholesterol
- Irregular heartbeat
- Liver issues
- Irritability and mood changes
- Decreased breast size
- Hair loss
- Acne
- Weight gain

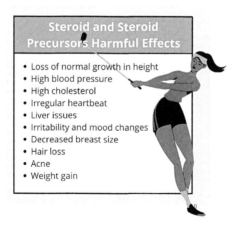

Human growth hormone
- Acromegaly (swelling of hands and feet, joint pain, dental problems, retention of fluid, and sweating)
- Heart damage
- Diabetes
- High blood pressure

- Osteoporosis
- High cholesterol

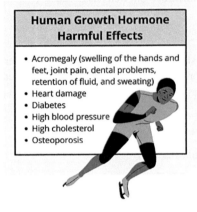

Amphetamines and stimulants
- High blood pressure
- Heart attack
- Shortness of breath
- Stroke
- Dizziness
- Anxiety
- Heat intolerance

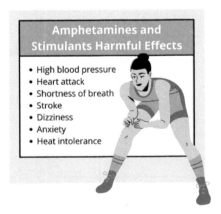

Creatine
- Nausea
- Abdominal pain
- Kidney damage

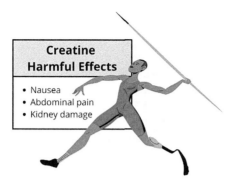

HOW BIG IS THE PED PROBLEM?

It is difficult to determine how large the problem is because people using PEDs are often not truthful in surveys. There are many studies estimating rates of 5–12% high schoolers using some sort of banned PED by grade 12.[2] This data often includes all students. It is known that males tend to have higher rates of usage, and sports that require more short bursts of strength usually have higher rates.

WHAT ARE THE RED FLAGS OF SOMEONE USING PEDs?

There are several things to watch for:

- Changes in behavior (irritability, increased aggressiveness)
- Increase in acne
- Needle marks
- Smaller breasts in women
- Excessive body hair growth
- Weight gain
- Muscle growth

PEDs RED Flags

▶ Changes in behavior (irritability and/or increased aggressiveness)

▶ Increase in acne

▶ Needle marks

▶ Smaller breasts in women

▶ Excessive body hair growth

▶ Weight gain

▶ Muscle growth

WHAT CAN PARENTS AND OTHERS DO TO PREVENT PED USE?

First, realize that if a teen uses PEDs, it is not always the fault of the parent. Most parents are surprised to find out that their children are using PEDs. Many teens feel a lot of internal pressure at baseline. Pressure from outside sources such as coaches or parents may play a part in their decision to take a banned substance. Encourage a fun and fitness approach. Discuss ethics in sports and fair play. Watch any purchases of supplements and read the labels to see what an energy drink or other performance product contains.

WHAT SHOULD BE DONE WHEN AN ATHLETE IS ON PEDs?

If an athlete is suspected of using PEDs, talk to them. Ask them why and discuss risks and benefits calmly. Discuss long-term repercussions. Encourage them to stop immediately. Make a physician appointment to discuss. Talking to the coach may be beneficial, especially as the coach may not know and there may be others on the team using. Most coaches emphatically discourage use of PEDs. But, if a coach is not helpful, speak to an athletic director.

Let's switch gears to another issue of nutrition intake.

WHAT ARE THE COMMON EATING DISORDERS?

The *Diagnostic and Statistical Manual of Mental Disorders* (DSM-5) defines several different eating disorders in the general population. Common disorders include anorexia nervosa, bulimia nervosa, and binge eating disorder. When there is solid evidence or even strong suspicion of any of these disorders, it is imperative that a treatment team communicates and works together to help the athlete progress in treatment and remission of the condition.

Anorexia Nervosa

Anorexia nervosa is a condition of significantly low BMI due to conscious restriction of food and energy intake. People with this disorder will have a fear of gaining weight even though they are in a malnourished state, along with a distorted body image and inability to recognize the seriousness of their current body state. It is more common in females than males, and onset is typically late adolescence to early adulthood.

The DSM-5 criteria for a diagnosis of anorexia nervosa include:

1. Restriction of energy intake relative to requirements leading to a significantly low body weight in the context of age, sex, developmental trajectory, and physical health. (Significantly low weight is defined as a body weight that is less than minimally normal for adults or, for children and adolescents, less than that minimally expected.)
2. Intense fear of gaining weight or becoming fat, even though underweight.

3. Disturbance in the way in which one's body weight or shape is experienced, undue influence of body weight or shape on self-evaluation, or denial of the seriousness of the current low body weight.Anorexia nervosa can be further categorized into two subtypes: restricting type and binge eating/purging type. Restriction type is restriction of energy intake in the absence of binging and purging. Binge eating/purging type requires regular engagement in either binge eating or purging. Furthermore, the severity of anorexia is based on BMI, with mild (BMI greater than or equal to 17 kg/m^2), moderate (BMI 16–16.99 kg/m^2), severe (BMI 15–15.99 kg/m^2), and extreme (BMI less than 15 kg/m^2).

There are many warning signs of anorexia. Physical signs include constipation, abdominal upset, lightheadedness, dizziness, cold intolerance, muscle weakness, fatigue, amenorrhea (loss of menstrual cycles), cavities, swelling of salivary glands, fine hair over body, and poor immune system function. Many of these symptoms are not specific and a detailed evaluation may need to be done by a physician.

Behavioral and emotional signs of anorexia include weight loss, refusal to eat foods, dressing in layers for warmth, feelings of being "fat", constant need to exercise in order to justify eating, irritability, and need for control over all calories taken in. Some methods used to control calorie intake include calorie counting, portion control, and purging methods including self-induced vomiting and use of diuretics ("water pills") or laxatives. It is important to be aware that some of the seemingly normal activities may be clues to a deeper issue.

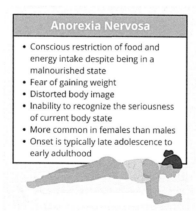

Anorexia Nervosa
- Conscious restriction of food and energy intake despite being in a malnourished state
- Fear of gaining weight
- Distorted body image
- Inability to recognize the seriousness of current body state
- More common in females than males
- Onset is typically late adolescence to early adulthood

BULIMIA NERVOSA

Similar to anorexia nervosa, bulimia nervosa is a condition that occurs most commonly in adolescent females and includes inappropriate compensatory behaviors to prevent weight gain.

The DSM-5 criteria for a diagnosis of bulimia nervosa include:

1. Recurrent episodes of binge eating. An episode of binge eating is characterized by both of the following:
   a. Eating, in a discrete period of time (e.g., within any 2-hour period), an
      amount of food that is definitely larger than most people would eat dur-
      ing a similar period of time and under similar circumstances.
   b. A sense of lack of control over overeating during the episode (e.g., a feel-
      ing that one cannot stop eating or control what or how much one is eating).
2. Recurrent inappropriate compensatory behavior to prevent weight gain,
   such as self-induced vomiting, misuse of laxatives, diuretics, or other medications, fasting, or excessive exercise.
3. The binge eating and inappropriate compensatory behaviors both occur, on
   average, at least once a week for three months.
4. Self-evaluation is unduly influenced by body shape and weight.
5. The disturbance does not occur exclusively during episodes of anorexia
   nervosa.[3]

There are many warning signs of bulimia. Behaviors include weight loss, dieting,
control of food, binge eating, trips to the bathroom after meals, odor of vomit, laxative use, food rituals, skipping meals, extreme fad dieting, hoarding of food, drinking
excessive non-caloric beverages, lots of mints or gum, excessive exercise, swelling
cheeks, calluses on hands, dental issues, withdrawal, bloating, and mood swings.
Physical signs include fluctuations in weight, gastrointestinal complaints, concentration problems, anemia, thyroid problems, low heart rate, dizziness, fainting, cold
intolerance, sleep problems, fine hair on body, weakness, menstrual abnormalities,
poor wound healing, and lowered immune function.

Bulimia Nervosa

- Inappropriate compensatory measures
  to prevent weight gain (self-induced
  vomiting; misuse of laxatives, diuretics
  or other medications; fasting;
  excessive exercise)
- Distorted body image
- Occurs most commonly in adolescent
  females

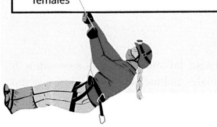

BINGE EATING DISORDER

Binge eating disorder is characterized by repeated episodes of large volumes of eating, feeling of loss of control, guilt, and purging. This is the most common eating disorder.

The DSM-5 criteria for a diagnosis of binge eating disorder include

1. Recurrent episodes of binge eating. An episode of binge eating is characterized by both of the following:
   a. Eating, in a discrete period of time (e.g., within any 2-hour period), an amount of food that is definitely larger than what most people would eat in a similar period of time under similar circumstances.
   b. A sense of lack of control over eating during the episode (e.g., a feeling that one cannot stop eating or control what or how much one is eating).
2. The binge eating episodes are associated with three (or more) of the following:
   a. Eating much more rapidly than normal.
   b. Eating until feeling uncomfortably full.
   c. Eating large amounts of food when not feeling physically hungry.
   d. Eating alone because of feeling embarrassed by how much one is eating.
   e. Feeling disgusted with oneself, depressed, or very guilty afterward.
3. Marked distress regarding binge eating is present.
4. The binge eating occurs, on average, at least once a week for 3 months.
5. The binge eating is not associated with the recurrent use of inappropriate compensatory behaviors (e.g., purging) as in bulimia nervosa and does not occur exclusively during the course of bulimia nervosa or anorexia nervosa.

Warning signs of binge eating disorder are similar to other eating disorders. Emotional and behavior signs include evidence of binge eating, extreme fad dieting, fear of eating in public, hoarding food, withdrawal, concern with weight and shape, food rituals, and low self-esteem. Physical signs include fluctuations in weight, gastrointestinal symptoms, and difficulty concentrating.

Binge Eating Disorder
- Repeated episodes of large volumes of eating, a feeling of loss of control, guilt, and purging
- Occurs, on average, at least once a week for three months
- Marked distress regarding binge eating is present
- Most common eating disorder

ORTHOREXIA

Orthorexia was not included in the latest classification of disorders, although it has been in the past and an awareness of the disorder is important. Orthorexia is an obsession with healthy eating. In general, healthy eating is positive, but when an obsession arises the athletes may become so fixated that it affects their well-being. This is often seen in individuals with obsessive compulsive disorder. Orthorexia shares some characteristics with anorexia as both involve restrictive issues.

Warning signs of orthorexia include checking labels, concern about ingredients, cutting out food groups, unusual interest in what others are eating, and showing stress when certain foods are not offered.

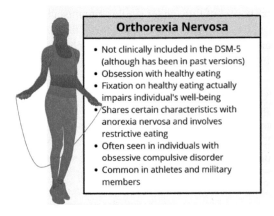

Orthorexia Nervosa

- Not clinically included in the DSM-5 (although has been in past versions)
- Obsession with healthy eating
- Fixation on healthy eating actually impairs individual's well-being
- Shares certain characteristics with anorexia nervosa and involves restrictive eating
- Often seen in individuals with obsessive compulsive disorder
- Common in athletes and military members

OTHER SPECIFIED FEEDING OR EATING DISORDERS

Another medical diagnosis is other specified feeding or eating disorders. It is used when there is a disorder present but the athlete doesn't fit criteria of the previously described eating disorders.

Long-term consequences of eating disorders include loss of menstrual cycle, loss of bone density, stress fractures, muscle wasting, brain atrophy, depression, impaired concentration, irritability, and electrolyte imbalances that can cause fatal heart abnormalities.

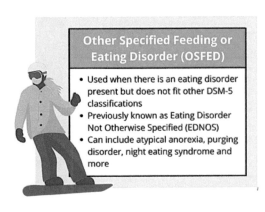

Other Specified Feeding or Eating Disorder (OSFED)

- Used when there is an eating disorder present but does not fit other DSM-5 classifications
- Previously known as Eating Disorder Not Otherwise Specified (EDNOS)
- Can include atypical anorexia, purging disorder, night eating syndrome and more

WHAT IS THE PREVALENCE OF EATING DISORDERS?

Eating disorders, such as the ones described here, are common in our society. The lifetime prevalence of anorexia nervosa is estimated to be 0.9% in women and 0.3% in men. The lifetime prevalence of bulimia nervosa is estimated to be 1.5% in women and 0.5% in men whereas the lifetime prevalence of binge eating disorder is 3.5% in women and 2.0% among men. While these prevalences seem low, threshold and subthreshold eating disorders are among the most common disorders in adolescent and young adult females. In fact, research suggests that the lifetime rate of anorexia nervosa in this group is 1.4%–2.0%, 1.1%–3.0% for subthreshold anorexia nervosa, 1.1%–4.6% for bulimia nervosa, 2.0%–5.4% for subthreshold bulimia nervosa, 0.2%–1.5% for binge eating disorder, and 1.6% for subthreshold eating disorder.[4]

Ironically, individuals with binge eating disorder often show high rates of obesity in the future. Another risk of eating disorders is that they often are left untreated. It is estimated that only 20%–50% of individuals who suffer from an eating disorder seek treatment, and only 30%–50% of those who receive treatment have a lasting recovery.[5]

While anyone can suffer from an eating disorder, it has been shown that athletes are more likely to develop one. There have been a variety of studies that have researched this concept. One had 522 female athletes and 448 female nonathletes complete an eating disorder questionnaire, undergo a clinical examination, and be interviewed. This study found that 18% of the athletes were diagnosed with eating disorders compared to only 5% of the nonathlete group. The study also found that the athletes tended to underreport disordered eating symptoms compared to the nonathlete group. There have been other studies that have found similar results. There is also a greater division in the frequency of eating disorders within different sports, with lean sports tending to have higher rates of disordered eating. A 2004 study by Sundgot-Borgen found there was a prevalence of disordered eating in aesthetic sports of 42%, in endurance sports of 24%, in technical sports of 17%, and in ball sports of 16%.[5]

Eating disorders appear in both male and female athletes, but they have been shown to be more common on the female side. Both sexes suffer from disordered eating and the problems that come with it. This was shown in a study where, of those surveyed, 20% of female athletes and 8% of male athletes qualified as having an eating disorder. These results were significantly different from the 9% of female controls and 0.5% of male controls who had an eating disorder. Male sports also appear to follow the general trend seen in female athletics where sports where the athletes are expected to be leaner have a higher prevalence of disordered eating.[6] Overall, athletes suffer at a higher rate from disordered eating than the general population does, and both sexes can be influenced by these disorders. But the group that is most afflicted is female athletes. This problem is so extreme that Lauren Fleshmen, a professional runner who has suffered from RED-S and disordered eating herself, reports that over one-third of Division 1 NCAA female athletes exhibit risk factors for anorexia nervosa.[7]

College female athletes are one of the most at-risk groups and have some of the highest occurrences of eating disorders. But this isn't a problem that only starts in college. Disordered eating can increase the likelihood of a female athlete developing RED-S, which is caused by insufficient caloric intake (such as disordered eating) and can lead to reduced energy, irregular menstrual cycles, and low bone density. RED-S can influence any individual but previous research has shown that this syndrome can arise in high school. An observational study of 170 female athletes, from eight different sports and six different schools in southern California, discovered the appearance of RED-S. It was reported that 18.2% of the athletes met the criteria for disordered eating, 23.5% for menstrual irregularity, and 21.8% for low bone mass. RED-S and eating disorders have dangerous health implications and decrease athletic performance. They are most common in female athletes and appear at the college level, but also in the younger age groups. It is important to understand these disorders and educate individuals to prevent future development and provide athletes with the support they need.[8]

HOW DO SOCIETIAL IDEALS CONTRIBUTE?

Unfortunately, our society perpetuates this image of an ideal female body. This is not new to our current generation. For most of history a woman's duty was to be attractive enough to get a husband, and body ideals followed this intention.[9] Several articles in the 1890s documented the effects of corsets, which included diminished lung capacity, digestive difficulties, rib abnormalities, and even heart palpitations.[10,11] These ideals are now well engrained in our society, even if people do not associate them with a marital duty. A survey done in 2017 showed that 87.9% of adolescent girls were concerned about their bodies.[12]

The SPRING Forward program discusses these ideals for what they are—antiquated, hurtful, misogynistic, and damaging. With the creation of photoshop and other editing devices, the images portrayed by media are not realistic. Many teens cannot achieve this body type without using damaging restrictive eating. They feel the pressure to look ideal and subsequently they feel they are never good enough when they do not duplicate the unrealistic bodies seen in the media.

In addition, many sports have body type ideals. Runners are expected to be very thin, yet some elite runners have muscular legs that appear bigger than the stereotype. Swimmers face similar issues with big muscular shoulders. In sports that require muscular strength, females often face disparaging remarks, as though they should concentrate on having smaller arms or legs.

Females also face many contradictory situations. Media shows them that they need to look like an "ideal" body. Team uniforms often show more skin than athletes desire, especially in sports like volleyball, handball, running, gymnastics, and swimming. Yet, females are told to cover their bodies so that they do not tempt males, as though a male's control of their desires is the fault of a female. None of this pressure is appropriate for adolescent females, or for that matter, adult females. For many athletes in the program, finding confidence to dress as they want and feel comfortable with their body type is a huge issue. The program focuses on increasing body image flexibility, which can be thought of as the ability to be confident in one's body regardless of the size or shape.

HOW IS AN EATING DISORDER DIAGNOSED?

It can be difficult to diagnose an eating disorder. Many times, teens will lie about their eating habits. There are questionnaires and screening methods. A physician will do a thorough history and physical exam. Tests may include electrolytes; kidney, thyroid and liver function tests; any other tests of possible deficiency; and an electrocardiogram.

HOW IS AN EATING DISORDER TREATED?

Treatment of eating disorders is complicated. The athlete may need help from a physician, psychologist, dietitian, school officials, teachers, and coaching staff.

There may be a need for treatment of the physical issues. Examples include correcting electrolyte disturbances and vitamin and mineral deficiencies. Sometimes there are complications during refeeding which require medical attention.

Hormonal imbalances may need to be addressed. Some physicians will prescribe oral contraceptives to help replace estrogen. It should be noted that oral contraceptives do not treat the underlying cause and do not necessarily help with bone density.

Psychological help is almost always needed. Therapy may include individual therapy or family therapy or both. Sometimes medication for issues such as depression or anxiety are useful. Psychological treatment may be necessary if there are other substance abuse issues in combination with the eating disorder.

Goals often include intake of adequate nutrition; obtaining a healthy weight; stopping binge eating, vomiting, and laxative abuse; and reducing excessive exercise. Many times, a return to sport includes maintaining some of these minimum goals.

There will be a need to monitor for months to years depending on the situation. It is not uncommon for an athlete to relapse, especially if they were hesitant to be diagnosed.

WHAT SHOULD I DO IF I SEE RED FLAGS IN AN ATHLETE?

In the event of warning signs, please get help. Schools in this program are encouraged to have a leader with resources to help. Talking to the athlete and their parents is a good start. Encourage them to see their physician for help. Some schools have a path in place for these issues already. There is a national helpline available at 1-800-931-2237. If the athlete is in a crisis mode, please call 911 or go to the nearest emergency department.

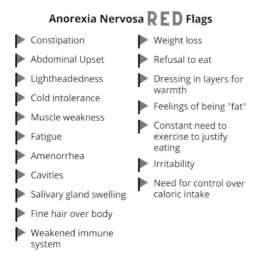

Anorexia Nervosa RED Flags

- Constipation
- Abdominal Upset
- Lightheadedness
- Cold intolerance
- Muscle weakness
- Fatigue
- Amenorrhea
- Cavities
- Salivary gland swelling
- Fine hair over body
- Weakened immune system
- Weight loss
- Refusal to eat
- Dressing in layers for warmth
- Feelings of being "fat"
- Constant need to exercise to justify eating
- Irritability
- Need for control over caloric intake

Bulimia Nervosa R E D Flags

▶ Fluctuations in weight   ▶ Weight loss

▶ Gastrointestinal issues   ▶ Dieting

▶ Concentration issues   ▶ Control of food

▶ Anemia   ▶ Trips to the bathroom
                                    after meals
▶ Thyroid problems
                                  ▶ Odor of vomit
▶ Low heart rate
                                  ▶ Laxative use
▶ Dizziness and fainting
                                  ▶ Food rituals
▶ Cold intolerance
                                  ▶ Caloric intake control
▶ Fine hair over body
                                  ▶ Excessive non-caloric
▶ Sleep problems   beverage intake or
                                    gum/mints
▶ Menstrual irregularities
                                  ▶ Calluses on hands
▶ Poor wound healing

Binge Eating Disorder R E D Flags

▶ Fluctuations in weight

▶ Gastrointestinal issues

▶ Concentration issues

▶ Extreme fad dieting

▶ Fear of eating in public

▶ Hoarding food

▶ Emotional withdrawal

▶ Concern with weight and shape

▶ Food rituals

▶ Low self-esteem

Orthorexia R E D Flags

▶ Constantly checking food labels

▶ Concern over ingredients

▶ Cutting out food groups

▶ Unusual interest in what others
  are eating

▶ Showing stress when certain
  food options are not available

AN ATHLETE'S STORY: LaShonda

I lived two different lives. While competing in the shot put, I was in my sweet spot. I started as a freshman. I had done wrestling and was strong. I lifted weights and took pride in my strength. I kept getting better and better throughout high school. My athletic life was amazing.

But there was a dark side. I hated my body. Some of the boys on the football team told me I was bigger than their linebackers. I went to the bathroom and cried. I knew I needed to be muscular to be good at shot put, but the insults hurt deeply. I couldn't look in the mirror. I started wearing really big clothes in an effort to mask my large muscles. People asked me if I was a lesbian. I wasn't but I was insulted that they made assumptions based on my muscular look. I didn't date in high school. I skipped prom and all social events. There was no way I was going to wear a cute dress and show all my large muscles. I became a complete hermit. Nobody spoke to me at school. At times I felt so alone, I thought about ending it all. But I did still enjoy the shot put and that kept me going.

I received a scholarship for college. I learned to be more comfortable with myself. I hung out with people who were positive. I made many friends lifting weights. Slowly, I came out of my shell. I became a little more social and met a guy I liked. He admired my muscular body and he lifted also. After college, we started doing body building together and eventually got married. I wish I had the confidence in high school to ignore the haters. I worry about girls who don't have something to keep them going.

CITATIONS

1. White, Nicole D, and James Noeun. "Performance-Enhancing Drug Use in Adolescence." *American Journal of Lifestyle Medicine*, 2016 Nov. 29; 11(2): 122–124. https://doi.org/10.1177/1559827616680593
2. Elflein, John. "Adolescent Drug Use in the U.S.—Statistics & Facts." *Statista*, February 15, 2022. Assessed June 27, 2022.
3. American Psychiatric Association. *Diagnostic and Statistical Manual of Mental Disorders* (5th ed.); 2013. https://doi.org/10.1176/appi.books.9780890425596
4. Hudson, James, Eva Hiripi, Harrison Pope, and Ronald Kessler. "The Prevalence and Correlates of Eating Disorders in the National Comorbidity Survey Replication." *Science Direct*, February 1, 2007.
5. Stice, Eric. *The Body Project*. New York: Oxford University Press; 2007.
6. Joy, Elizabeth, Andrea Kussman, and Aurelia Nattiv. "2016 Update on Eating Disorders in Athletes: A Comprehensive Narrative Review with a Focus on Clinical Assessment and Management." *British Journal of Sports Medicine*, December 7, 2015.
7. Fleshman, Lauren. "I Changed My Body for My Sport. No Girl Should." *New York Times*, November 16, 2019.
8. Nichols, Jeanne, Mitchell Rauh, and Mandra Lawson. "Prevalence of the Female Athlete Triad Syndrome among High School Athletes." *JAMA Pediatrics*, February, 2006.

9. Parker R. The Female Body and Body Image: A Historical Perspective. In: Parker R. *Women, Doctors and Cosmetic Surgery: Negotiating the "Normal" Body.* London: Palgrave Macmillan; 2009: 25–37.

10. Death from Tight Lacing. *Lancet.* 1890; 135(3485): 1316.

11. Effects of Tight-Lacing. *Lancet.* 1892; 139(3568): 151–152.

12. Bullot A, Cave L, Fildes J, Hall S, Plummer J. *Mission Australia Youth Survey Report 2017.* https://www.missionaustralia.com.au/publications/youth-survey/746-youth-survey-2017-report/file. Accessed August 14, 2019.

6 Relative Energy Deficiency in Sport (RED-S)

Kathryn Vidlock

Rocky Vista University, Parker, CO, USA

Catherine Liggett

University of Colorado School of Medicine, Aurora, CO, USA

CONTENTS

WORDS TO KNOW

AMENORRHEA   Loss of menses.

FEMALE ATHLETE TRIAD   Older term consisting of disordered eating and lower energy availability, irregular menstrual cycles and hormonal imbalances, and decreased bone density and osteoporosis.

MENSES   Menstrual cycles or periods.

RELATIVE ENERGY DEFICIENCY IN SPORT (RED-S)   A syndrome caused by energy deficiency, potentially impacting metabolism, hormones, menstrual function, bone health, immunity, protein synthesis, and heart function.

DOI: 10.1201/b23228-6

WHY DOES ENERGY BALANCE MATTER?

Energy balance is very important to female athletes' body regulation. When female athletes do not consume enough calories, they experience an energy deficiency. Sometimes this happens with restrictive eating, illness-causing malabsorption, or true eating disorders. Regardless, an energy deficit occurs, affecting the body's ability to regulate itself and perform well.

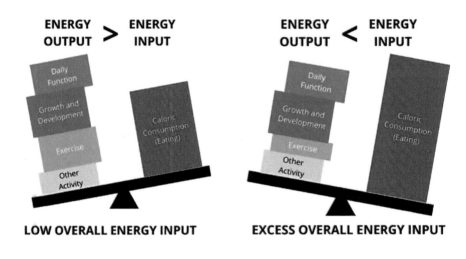

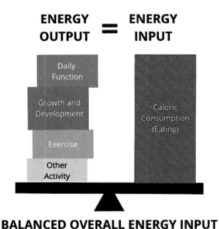

WHAT IS THE FEMALE ATHLETE TRIAD?

For many years, professionals have talked about the female athlete triad. The triad concept is simply a way of illustrating what happens within the spectrum of low energy availability. It is an older model but some are familiar with it. The energy deficiency leads to irregular or missed menses and hormonal dysfunction. Eventually, this leads to decreased bone density and osteoporosis.[1]

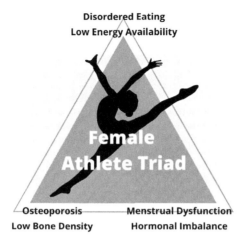

It is now known that energy deficiency affects a multitude of body systems. Areas affected include metabolism, bone health, psychological/emotional, and endocrine (hormonal including menstrual), immune, gastrointestinal, and cardiovascular systems. This has led to a new definition of relative energy deficiency syndrome.[2]

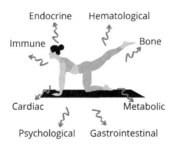

Some athletes simply eat too little because of a fad diet or because they believe it will make them faster or a better athlete. There are some athletes who may benefit from weight loss, and they may need nutritional counseling to do it in a healthy manner. Athletes who are at an appropriate weight do not need to lose weight and may, in fact, have worse performance if they lose weight. Other athletes restrict their eating in a manner consistent with an eating disorder. The difference between healthy eating and restrictive eating can be hard to differentiate at times. Athletes losing weight or exhibiting symptoms of fatigue or overtraining are at risk for having RED-S.

When an athlete takes in fewer calories than expended, this results in a negative energy balance. In female athletes, the symptoms affect hormones; symptoms can include restrictive eating (or eating disorders), osteoporosis (decreased bone density), and amenorrhea (loss of periods). Some athletes only have one or a few of the symptoms, while others may have many. Athletes in certain sports where there is an expectation of lean bodies are more at risk (running, swimming, gymnastics).

WHAT IS THE CAUSE OF RED-S?

The cause is the underlying energy deficiency. Energy availability is the energy intake minus energy cost of exercise. An average adult needs 45 kcal/kg FFM/day to create an energy balance. The true amount for adolescent athletes is not fully known and may be different. For practical purposes, most studies use the 45 kcal/kg FFM/day. A lower intake creates an energy deficit.[3]

HOW DOES THIS CORRELATE WITH EATING DISORDERS?

Eating disorders are at one end of a spectrum with healthy eating at the opposite end. The official diagnostic criteria for eating disorders are covered in Chapter 5, but the types include anorexia nervosa, bulimia nervosa, binge disorder, and unspecified disorders. Eating disorders, unintentional undereating, and other disorders can all lead to an energy deficit.

SPECTRUM OF EATING BEHAVIOR

Intuitive Eating	Disordered Eating	Eating Disorder
• Follows hunger cues	• Restriction of food intake to control weight/shape	• Extreme restriction of food
• Eats all food groups		• Focus on eating negatively influences other aspects of life
• Finds eating to be a pleasurable experience	• Follows rigid food rules (counting calories/macros, cutting out certain food groups, intermittent fasting)	
• Lacks shame or guilt surrounding eating		• Extreme guilt over eating "bad" foods
• Allows for indulgences	• Feels shameful about breaking "food rules"	• Purging (vomiting, laxatives) and/or binging
• Defines food neutrally	• Labels food as either "good" or "bad"	• Exercises through injuries and illnesses out of fear of gaining weight during time off
• Exercises for health and enjoyment	• Uses exercise as means to justify eating or as solely a way to burn calories	• Over-exercises and refuses recovery days

WHAT KINDS OF PROBLEMS ARE SEEN IN THE BODY?

Almost every body system can be affected by prolonged energy deficiency. One of the biggest is the endocrine system. With an energy deficiency, less gonadotrophin-releasing hormones (GnRH, a hormone) are released from the hypothalamus (a gland in the brain). This leads to less luteinizing hormone (LH) and follicle-stimulating hormone (FSH) (hormones regulating menses) being released from the pituitary gland. Subsequently less estrogen and progesterone are released, which leads to a loss of menses.

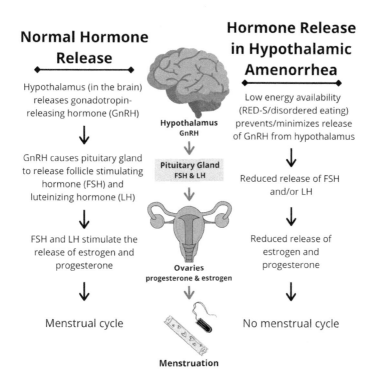

Loss of menses may be a warning sign. This can be difficult to assess in teenagers because many females will have somewhat irregular cycles in their early teens. Primary amenorrhea is when a female doesn't start having their menstrual cycle. Secondary amenorrhea is when a female has at least one cycle and then the cycles stop. Both conditions are concerning. Sometimes female athletes do not start their periods by their late teens and believe there is no issue simply because they haven't started, but that is not the case. Missing menstrual cycles may seem convenient for high school athletes, but there are negative consequences. Other irregularities such as light bleeding may occur with hormonal changes as well, complicating this further. Eventually, this may affect fertility.

Estrogen helps calcium deposition into the bone. Progesterone helps with estrogen function. Other hormones play a role, including IgF-1. The mechanism is complex, but it is established that an energy deficiency leads to a decrease in many hormones responsible for bone health and subsequently low bone density. If serious this can cause osteoporosis and stress fractures. Low estrogen can lead to heart problems, low energy, and mood disorders. Long-term effects can include lifelong osteoporosis.[4]

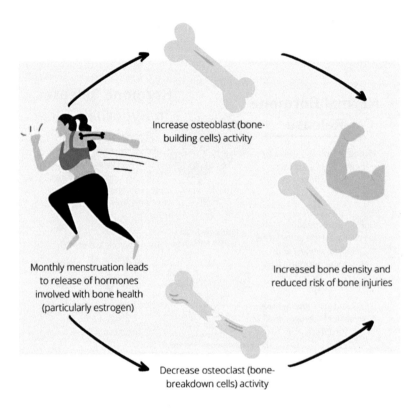

Increase osteoblast (bone-building cells) activity

Increased bone density and reduced risk of bone injuries

Monthly menstruation leads to release of hormones involved with bone health (particularly estrogen)

Decrease osteoclast (bone-breakdown cells) activity

Lack of nutrients may lead to iron deficiency, which leads to anemia or a decrease in hemoglobin, which is needed to carry oxygen to organs. Eating disorders may lead to abnormalities in the electrolytes in the bloodstream.

Cardiac problems include slow heart rate (bradycardia), larger increases in heart rate with activity, low blood pressure, and disturbances in heart rhythm. Heart rhythm disorders can be fatal. The gastrointestinal system may also be affected. The usual symptoms are slow digestion and constipation. Some athletes may also feel bloated.

Psychological disorders are common. Eating disorders are the obvious issue, but often depression and anxiety are seen. Mood swings and irritability are common as well. Athletes may feel a brain fog sensation or decreased concentration.

Metabolism can slow down. Generation of protein decreases. There is a decrease in glucose usage and fat storage is used. Fatigue can set in and affect training. The immune system is affected, and the athlete may experience more viral illnesses.[5]

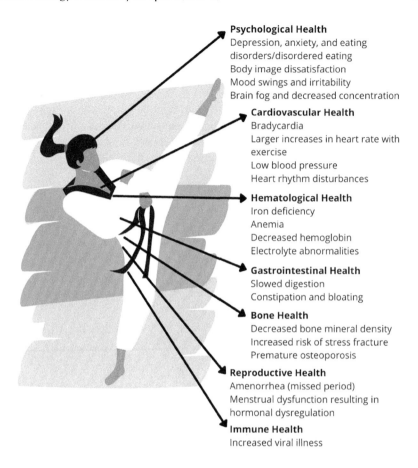

Psychological Health
Depression, anxiety, and eating
disorders/disordered eating
Body image dissatisfaction
Mood swings and irritability
Brain fog and decreased concentration

Cardiovascular Health
Bradycardia
Larger increases in heart rate with
exercise
Low blood pressure
Heart rhythm disturbances

Hematological Health
Iron deficiency
Anemia
Decreased hemoglobin
Electrolyte abnormalities

Gastrointestinal Health
Slowed digestion
Constipation and bloating

Bone Health
Decreased bone mineral density
Increased risk of stress fracture
Premature osteoporosis

Reproductive Health
Amenorrhea (missed period)
Menstrual dysfunction resulting in
hormonal dysregulation

Immune Health
Increased viral illness

ARE DIFFERENT RACES AFFECTED IN A DIFFERENT WAY?

At this time the vast majority of RED-S research has been done on European and European American female athletes. There is a lower prevalence of RED-S in African American females—although the lack of current research in this group may be contributory to this finding.[6] African American females have higher bone density in general, but it is not known if this plays a role in the decreased incidence. There is a large need for further research on racially diverse populations of female athletes.

HOW DO I KNOW IF AN ATHLETE HAS RED-S?

The screening for RED-S is very difficult. Even physicians, dietitians, and other professionals have difficulty. Athletes may lie about their caloric intake and not want to admit to restrictive eating. The instructors for this course should not hold themselves responsible for detecting eating disorders or RED-S. If they feel there are warning signs or an athlete wants further help, please refer to the resources in the back of the book or other local resources from the school.

HOW IS RED-S TREATED?

Treatment of RED-S is multifactorial and requires collaboration of physicians, psychologists, dietitians, coaches, athletic trainers, and school officials. Multiple aspects of RED-S need to be addressed, including the energy deficit, nutritional and psychological aspects, and any medical issues caused by the energy deficit.

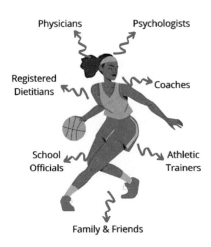

WHAT SHOULD BE THE PLAN IF RED FLAGS ARE PRESENT?

We encourage the leaders to have a plan in place for any athlete exhibiting red flag symptoms. This may involve notifying the guidance counselor, the school psychologist, coaches, and parents. It is helpful for the school to designate a SPRING Forward for Girls director. Each school has different resources so plans will vary. A sample plan may look like the following:

- Red flag issue identified.
- Meet with athlete and parents.
- Recommend evaluation with primary care physician and appropriate referrals to psychologists or specialists.
- Inform any appropriate school personnel, such as coaches, nurses, psychologists, and athletic trainers.

Please keep in mind the confidentiality needs of athletes when communicating with appropriate individuals.

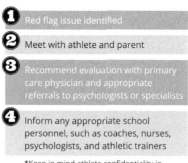

1 Red flag issue identified

2 Meet with athlete and parent

3 Recommend evaluation with primary care physician and appropriate referrals to psychologists or specialists

4 Inform any appropriate school personnel, such as coaches, nurses, psychologists, and athletic trainers

*Keep in mind athlete confidentiality in communicating with certain individuals

---

AN ATHLETE'S STORY: Shayla

My family is really tall. I felt like the odd one out because I was always short in grade school. I went to a cheer camp in fifth grade and had so much fun. I was a flyer and loved being up high. Then puberty hit me. I grew like a weed. I kept doing some strength and core training for cheer. I was also pretty quiet and loved to read. I was an A student and loved math. The other cheerleaders called me the smart girl or nerd. But they did it lovingly so I didn't care. They knew I was the one who would tutor them if needed.

By freshman year of high school I was 5′5″ and weighed 125. My cheer coach told me I was too big to be a flyer anymore and made me a base. I was so embarrassed and had some tears in practice that day. Some of the girls were trying to help and offered diet tips. They drank lots of water and diet pop. They ate carrots and lettuce and grapes for meals. I used their tips briefly, but I didn't like being hungry. I hated my body. I went through cycles of trying new diets (keto, gluten free, etc.) and then hating the diet and not caring what I ate or weighed. My weight went from 125 down to 112 and back up to 130, over and over depending on my current diet.

The worst day was when some of the football team asked why I wasn't the one up in the air anymore. One of my teammates told them it was because I had gotten too big. They called me chubby and laughed. My teammate yelled at them, but the damage was done. Chubs was my nickname among the football players. The irony of the overweight football players calling a girl with a normal BMI chubby was lost on me for many years. I believed them completely and I knew I would never date. I avoided mirrors. I became more of a loner and didn't go out with friends. My cheer friends tried to be helpful. They told me I was a great base and that it was great that I had thick legs. That statement hurt even though they meant it to be helpful. Our uniforms had short skirts that showed my thick thighs. I loved the cold days when we wore pants.

By the time I graduated high school I was 5'9". I did not cheer my senior year. I told people I wanted to concentrate on my AP classes, but the truth was that I didn't want to be called chubby anymore. I took up running to try and lose weight but it did not work and just made me more hungry. I hated running anyway.

I went to a local state university and decided to try cheer there. Again, I was a base but nobody called me chubby. I cheered for 2 years, but my heart was not in it. I missed being a flyer. I went to a physician on campus to get advice on how to lose weight. He told me my BMI was on the low side of normal and advised against dieting. He asked me if I had an eating disorder and I said no. But I started wondering. I looked up some information and I really didn't fit neatly into any category. But I was not happy with my body. My thighs were so big and muscular.

I graduated with a degree in international communication and traveled a lot. I was afraid to try new foods because I didn't know how many calories or fat or even what the ingredients were. Over the years, I have expanded my diet but I still struggle with feeling chubby occasionally. I still have larger thighs than most women my age.

I wish I had a program in my high school that taught body positivity as this program does. It is important for girls of all sizes to be accepted. Schools need to educate coaches and athletes on issues of eating and body image. I hope that one day it will become the norm for girls of all sizes to participate in activities and sports. I also hope it will become unacceptable for male athletes to make insensitive remarks about female's bodies.

CITATIONS

1. Nattiv A, Loucks AB, Manore MM, Sanborn CF, Sundgot-Borgen J, Warren MP. American College of Sports Medicine Position Stand. The Female Athlete Triad. *Med Sci Sports Exerc.* 2007 Oct;39(10):1867–1882. doi:10.1249/mss.0b013e318149f111. PMID: 17909417.

2. Mountjoy M, Sundgot-Borgen J, Burke L, et al. The IOC consensus statement: beyond the Female Athlete Triad—Relative Energy Deficiency in Sport (RED-S). *Br J Sports Med.* 2014;48:491–497.

3. Wasserfurth P, Palmowski J, Hahn A, Krüger K. Reasons for and Consequences of Low Energy Availability in Female and Male Athletes: Social Environment, Adaptations, and Prevention. *Sports Med Open.* 2020;6(1):44. Published 2020 Sep 10. doi:10.1186/s40798-020-00275-6.

4. Lambrinoudaki I, Papadimitriou D Pathophysiology of Bone Loss in the Female Athlete. *Ann N Y Acad Sci.* 2010;1205:45–50.

5. Hagmar M, Hirschberg AL, Berglund L, et al. Special Attention to the Weight-Control Strategies Employed by Olympic Athletes Striving for Leanness Is Required. *Clin J Sport Med.* 2008;18:5–9.

6. Pernick Y, Nichols JF, Rauh MJ, et al. Disordered Eating among a Multi-Racial/Ethnic Sample of Female High-School Athletes. *J Adolesc Health.* 2006; 38:689–695.

7 Information for Schools and Teams
Logistics

Kathryn Vidlock
Rocky Vista University, Parker, CO, USA

Catherine Liggett
University of Colorado School of Medicine, Aurora, CO, USA

CONTENTS

WORDS TO KNOW

RELATIVE ENERGY DEFICIENCY IN SPORT (RED-S) A syndrome caused by energy deficiency, potentially impacting metabolism, hormones, menstrual function, bone health, immunity, protein synthesis, and heart function.

SPRING FORWARD AMBASSADORS Student leaders who act as role models and peer leaders. They may lead the groups with proper training.

SPRING FORWARD FOR GIRLS DIRECTOR A specified individual at a school or district who is the main leader and helps facilitate the organization of the program

DOI: 10.1201/b23228-7

and may be of help with troubleshooting or aiding with athletes who exhibit red flag symptoms.

SPRING LEADER   Individuals who will facilitate the sessions. These may be coaches, teachers, alumni, or other interested individuals.

GENERAL INFORMATION

The past chapters have explained the history and need for interventions for teen female athletes for both improving body image and nutritional knowledge. This program is specifically designed for high school–age athletes. The level of knowledge and nutritional needs are slightly different than their college counterparts. This chapter goes over the practical aspects of implementing the three sessions and issues that may arise.

This course is three sessions long and the overall goal is to promote flexible thinking toward a positive body image and using nutrition for proper fueling.

WHAT SKILLS DOES A SESSION LEADER NEED?

There are no prerequisites for being a leader. Ideally, a leader would have some knowledge of the sport(s) in which the athletes compete. The leader should have a strong desire to promote healthy nutrition for fueling and a mindset for positive body image. Reading the background information in this book will provide the basic information needed to lead a session. The question arises about having female leaders for female athletes. That is left up to the schools and teams. In general, we have found that female athletes feel a little more comfortable opening up around female leaders; however, there are many males who would be extremely effective facilitators and should not be discouraged simply due to gender.

WHAT IS THE SPRING FORWARD FOR GIRLS DIRECTOR AND WHAT ARE THEIR RESPONSIBILITIES?

Ideally, each school will have a SPRING Forward for Girls director. This person may or may not lead sessions. Their usual responsibility would be to facilitate getting the necessary supplies (instruction books for leaders, copies of handouts) and helping find available space to meet and communicate with coaches and teams about the program. In addition, they should have identified resources in case an athlete exhibits red flag symptoms of an eating disorder or psychological issue. This director might be the athletic director, a coach, or other personnel at the school or district. The director doesn't need to be a SPRING leader. They are not expected to be an expert, but they should know how to get an athlete with red flags to appropriate help.

SPRING Ambassadors

- Peer leaders
- Act as role models
- Read nutrition and RED-S info
- NOT expected to be experts
- Might act as a liaison if an athlete is uncomfortable talking to an adult leader
- Should get a leader or the director involved if any red flags noticed
- Should not feel responsible for diagnosis or treatment of RED-s or eating disorders
- Use this as leadership experience on college applications

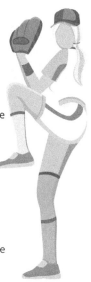

WHAT IS A SPRING LEADER?

A SPRING leader is just an adult responsible for the sessions. It may be the same person as the director or it may be a coach, teacher, or other responsible adult. They may lead a group if needed, but they are essentially an adult presence. At the college level and beyond it may not be necessary, but it is recommended to have one at the high school level.

WHAT ARE SPRING AMBASSADORS AND HOW MANY SHOULD WE HAVE?

SPRING Ambassadors are athletes who are peer leaders. They might lead and facilitate the groups, depending on the school's desire. They encourage and act as role models to their team. They are expected to read the background information, nutrition information, and RED-S information. More formal training may take place depending on the school. They are not expected to be experts. The leaders act as facilitators. They also may act as communication liaisons if an athlete is uncomfortable talking directly to an adult leader. If a SPRING Ambassador notices any red flags in an athlete they should get a leader or the director involved immediately. They should not feel responsible for any diagnosis or treatment of RED-S or eating disorders.

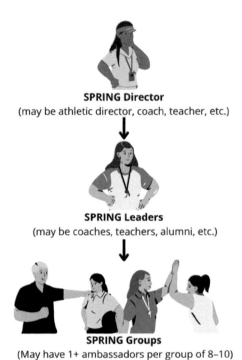

SPRING Director
(may be athletic director, coach, teacher, etc.)

SPRING Leaders
(may be coaches, teachers, alumni, etc.)

SPRING Groups
(May have 1+ ambassadors per group of 8–10)

WHAT ARE THE GOALS OF EACH SESSION?

Session 1 goals focus on getting the group talking and feeling comfortable. The session starts off with an ice breaker. The basics of nutrition and the changes needed in nutrition over the season are discussed, along with the basics of body image and media influences.

Session 2 goals are furthering knowledge on nutrition. We discuss recovery nutrition and fueling appropriately for competition and sport-specific nutrition needs. We continue to discuss positive body image issues.

Session 3 goals are cementing the positive body image and empowering the female athletes to make good decisions as well as understanding red flag behaviors in themselves and teammates.

One of the tools used is a positivity circle. One female athlete is in the middle and the others go around stating positive attributes of that athlete. Each athlete takes a turn in the middle. This may feel uncomfortable at first, but feedback is usually overwhelmingly positive. The overall idea is that it is much easier to give compliments than receive them.

WHAT ARE THE RED FLAGS A LEADER SHOULD WATCH FOR?

Group leaders, coaches, and parents should watch for red flags in female teenage athletes. Behavioral changes include obsession with food, calories, and weight;

avoidance of food-related activities; restrictive eating or binge eating; and frequent bathroom visits after meals. Physical changes may include excessive exercising, wearing baggy clothes, decreased weight or fluctuation in weight and body fat, stress fractures, hormonal abnormalities, loss of menstrual cycles, and increased growth of fine body hair. Psychological changes may include negativity about one's body, out-of-control feelings, and symptoms of depression and anxiety.[1] Most likely, a leader will not have to deal with any of these, however, they should be prepared if it arises.

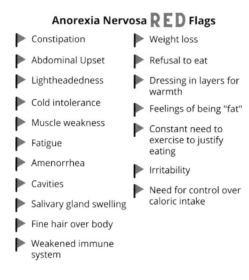

Anorexia Nervosa RED Flags

- Constipation
- Abdominal Upset
- Lightheadedness
- Cold intolerance
- Muscle weakness
- Fatigue
- Amenorrhea
- Cavities
- Salivary gland swelling
- Fine hair over body
- Weakened immune system

- Weight loss
- Refusal to eat
- Dressing in layers for warmth
- Feelings of being "fat"
- Constant need to exercise to justify eating
- Irritability
- Need for control over caloric intake

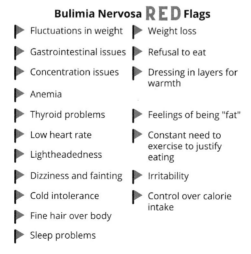

Bulimia Nervosa RED Flags

- Fluctuations in weight
- Gastrointestinal issues
- Concentration issues
- Anemia
- Thyroid problems
- Low heart rate
- Lightheadedness
- Dizziness and fainting
- Cold intolerance
- Fine hair over body
- Sleep problems

- Weight loss
- Refusal to eat
- Dressing in layers for warmth
- Feelings of being "fat"
- Constant need to exercise to justify eating
- Irritability
- Control over calorie intake

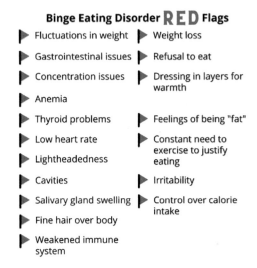

Binge Eating Disorder R E D Flags

- Fluctuations in weight
- Weight loss
- Gastrointestinal issues
- Refusal to eat
- Concentration issues
- Dressing in layers for warmth
- Anemia
- Thyroid problems
- Feelings of being "fat"
- Low heart rate
- Constant need to exercise to justify eating
- Lightheadedness
- Cavities
- Irritability
- Salivary gland swelling
- Control over calorie intake
- Fine hair over body
- Weakened immune system

Orthorexia R E D Flags

- Constantly checking food labels
- Concern over ingredients
- Cutting out food groups
- Unusual interest in what others are eating
- Showing stress when certain food options are not available

WHAT DO WE DO WHEN WE SEE RED FLAG SYMPTOMS?

It is recommended that every school have a plan in place for any athlete with red flag symptoms. This may be as simple as alerting a coach, athletic trainer, or athletic director. That responsible party will meet with the athlete and possibly parents, depending on age. A plan to address the situation will be made, including possible intervention with physician, dietitian, psychologist, or another specialist. Always remember confidentiality issues are of highest importance.

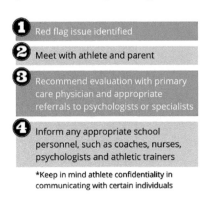

1. Red flag issue identified
2. Meet with athlete and parent
3. Recommend evaluation with primary care physician and appropriate referrals to psychologists or specialists
4. Inform any appropriate school personnel, such as coaches, nurses, psychologists and athletic trainers

*Keep in mind athlete confidentiality in communicating with certain individuals

TROUBLESHOOTING

Missed sessions Our approach is to allow girls to attend sessions even if they have missed a prior session. When possible, the group leader may choose to recap the previous session one on one with the participant.

Engagement At first the athletes may be hesitant to engage in the discussions. Usually they will warm to the idea by the end of the first session. The hardest part for the athletes is often the friendship circle. They will likely enjoy complimenting other athletes but will have difficulty being in the center. It will help to maintain eye contact with the athletes. If needed, leaders can call on specific participants or go around the circle answering questions. If needed, remind them of the confidentiality within the group and encourage respectful remarks, especially if a participant is revealing personal issues.

Breaking confidentiality If a participant shares personal information outside of the group, the leaders should address the situation both with the individual and the group. If serious enough, the athlete may be asked to leave the program.

Homework There is a minimal amount of homework after Sessions 1 and 2. We highly encourage the athletes to do the homework but allow and encourage them to keep participating if they do not. The athletes who complete the homework generally feel they have learned more than those who do not.

Differences in knowledge, mindset, and sport abilities There will naturally be athletes of different levels. There is also a difference in mindsets of various individuals. The mental toughness of athletes is quite variable in teenagers. There is some evidence that athletes with more mental toughness are able to make better lifestyle choices.[2] Female athletes tend to have less confidence, control, and self-esteem than males.[3] Mental toughness correlates with sport satisfaction, which is correlated to overall well-being and athletic performance.[3–5] In each group of female athletes, there will likely be varying levels of confidence, abilities, self-esteem, and well-being. Eating disorders, depression, anxiety, and other mental health issues may be present in small groups.

MONITORING SUCCESS

We encourage each school to elicit feedback for improvement. We generally use a simple format, either written or oral, asking what was most valuable and what could be improved. We also ask if they would recommend this to their athletic friends and why or why not. Some schools may choose to use questionnaires at the beginning and end for the athletes to compare their scores. Our recommendation would be the BI-AAQ as that measures body image flexibility. The questionnaires are optional and it will not impact learning to go without.

PREVIOUS RESULTS

The SPRING Forward program has been used in schools in Colorado. The study used body image flexibility scores to assess change. Body image flexibility can be thought of as the "ability to fully experience the present moment while engaging in behavior that is consistent with one's chosen values even when the present moment includes difficult emotions, thoughts, memories or body sensations".[6]

The cross-country/track team showed a statistically significant increase of 26.5% in body image flexibility. The cheer team showed an increase of 22.75%. Overall scores increased by 23.91%.[7]

AN ATHLETE'S STORY: Annette

I went out for tennis my freshman year because I was really overweight. Tennis was a no-cut sport at my school. I had never done anything athletic. My family wasn't into sports or outdoor activities. We were encouraged to do music and I played the oboe in band and was in choir. I had envisioned being skinny by the end of the season.

I was on the bottom end of the junior varsity team. I only played in two matches all year. Despite never missing a practice I only lost 2 pounds all season. How could that happen? I had also eaten anything I wanted—and junk food all the time.

Part of our health class that year was nutrition. I made a small bet with myself that if I could go 1 week without junk food, I would treat myself to a Blizzard at the end of the week. I made it and before I got the Blizzard, I decided to go for 2 weeks. I also decided to cut out fats. At the end of 2 weeks, I weighed myself. I had lost 7 pounds! I decided to skip the blizzard and go for 3 weeks. Week by week I lost weight. When it got hard, I would eat, then force myself to throw up or take laxatives. I prepared for Thanksgiving and other holidays by taking laxatives before the meal. Most of the time I restricted my eating. I skipped breakfast—told my parents I was eating at school. I skipped lunch by telling friends I had to go to classes to work. By dinner I was super hungry, but I ate the bare minimum to not arouse suspicion.

For the first time, I felt confident in my body. I bought short skirts and shorts. I became more social. Nobody called me fat anymore. If I could just try harder I could be as skinny as models.

One day in gym, I fainted. The school nurse asked me what I had eaten. I hadn't eaten for over 24 hours, but I lied. I told her it was time for my cycle, and she thought that was the cause. I hadn't had my cycle for months by that point.

That same week, my sister caught me throwing up in the bathroom. I tried to tell my parents I was just sick, but my mom didn't believe me. She took me to our physician. I was in the normal weight range for the first time in my life. I told my physician I didn't want to gain all the weight back. I was terrified of being fat. She told me she was happy I had lost weight, but she wanted me to do it in the right way. She referred me to a dietitian who specialized in eating disorders. I went to several sessions. I loved learning about the right way to eat and especially how to eat during my tennis season. I know she doesn't think she did anything special, but that dietitian saved me. My whole world changed after our sessions. She was so nice and gave me the straight facts and encouraged me to cheat on diets sometimes. She used to tease me and say—add sprinkles to the donuts, sweetie.

My senior year I was the lowest person to make the varsity team—BUT I MADE IT. I felt like a true athlete. Eating correctly left me with energy and a healthy feeling. The season was the most fun time in my high school years, even though we mostly lost.

I went to college and studied to be a dietitian. I work mostly with adults, but I occasionally get a chance to work with teen girls and I truly love it. The idea of doing more of this education in schools is way overdue. Take the opportunity to learn and be easy on yourselves. One of my favorite quotes is: "The best weight to lose is the weight of other people's opinion of you". Don't let society dictate your self-worth. You go, girls!

CITATIONS

1. Wells KR, Jeacocke NA, Appaneal R, et al. The Australian Institute of Sport (AIS) and National Eating Disorders Collaboration (NEDC) Position Statement on Disordered Eating in High Performance Sport. *Br J Sports Med.* 2020; 54 (21): 1247–1258. doi:10.1136/bjsports-2019-101813.

2. Stamp E, Crust L, Swann C. The Impact of Mental Toughness on Lifestyle Choices in University Students. *British Association of Sport and Exercise Science Annual Conference*, 2015.

3. Zeiger JS, Zeiger RS. Mental Toughness Latent Profiles in Endurance Athletes. *PLoS One.* 2018; 13(2): e0193071. Published 2018 Feb 23. doi:10.1371/journal.pone.0193071.

4. Reinboth M, Duda JL. Perceived Motivational Climate, Need Satisfaction and Indices of Well-Being in Team Sports: A Longitudinal Perspective. *Psychol Sport Exerc.* 2006; 7: 269–286.

5. Gillet N, Vallerand RJ, Amoura S, Baldes B. Influence of Coaches' Autonomy Support on Athletes' Motivation and Sport Performance: A Test of the Hierarchical Model of Intrinsic and Extrinsic Motivation. *Psychol Sport Exerc.* 2010; 11: 155–161.

6. Hayes SC, Luoma JB, Bond FW, Masuda A, Lillis J. Acceptance and Commitment Therapy: Model, Processes, and Outcomes. *Behav Res Ther.* 2006; 44(1): 1–25. doi:10.1016/j.brat.2005.06.006.

7. Vidlock K, Liggett C, Oberlag N. Improvement of Body Image Flexibility in Adolescent Female Athletes Undergoing Education about Nutrition and Body Image. *J Food Sci Nutr Res.* 5 (2022): 638–644.

8 Session Manual for Adolescent Athletes

Kathryn Vidlock

Rocky Vista University, Parker, CO, USA

Catherine Liggett

University of Colorado School of Medicine, Aurora, CO, USA

Nicole Oberlag

Claremont College, Claremont, CA, USA

CONTENTS

DOI: 10.1201/b23228-8

WORDS TO KNOW

RELATIVE ENERGY DEFICIENCY IN SPORT (RED-S)   A syndrome caused by energy deficiency, potentially impacting metabolism, hormones, menstrual function, bone health, immunity, protein synthesis, and heart function.

SESSION 1

Supplies—whiteboard or paper easel, markers, homework handout, training plates handout, the importance of breakfast handout, eating disorder questionnaire, if desired

Timing: Early in the season

Topic Areas

    I. Introduction (5 minutes)
   II. Group Rules and Expectations (5 minutes)
  III. Defining/Discussing Healthy Mindset and Body Image (20 minutes)
  IV. Nutrition for the Season (15 minutes)
   V. Homework—One nutrition goal and one mindset goal for positive change. Write down five things about your body and mindset that are helping your performance (5 minutes)
  VI. Conclusion (10 minutes)

INTRODUCTION (5 MINUTES)

Leaders introduce themselves briefly. Take about 30 seconds.

- *What are your personal interests and passions?*
- *What are your past areas of study?*
- *What made you want to do this project?*
- *Did you struggle with these issues as a high school athlete?*

Have the girls introduce themselves—they should share their name and one thing they like about their body or mindset.

Remind participants that this program is educational and they may participate to the extent they desire, including not participating at all. The athlete can also feel free to use their involvement in this program as part of their college application if they feel it is useful. Reinforce the fact that this school, district, coaches, and leadership endorse the goal of improved body image in all of its members.

There will be optional homework to do alongside attendance of three sessions. This homework is not required, but in exchange, athletes will benefit from improved nutrition and hopefully performance as well as lifelong health benefits. They will likely get more out of this program if they choose to complete the homework.

If using social media, also recommend following SPRING Forward social media accounts for more extensive information.

- Instagram: @spring_forward_girls
- Facebook: @springforwardgirls
- Website: springforwardgirls.com

GROUP RULES AND EXPECTATIONS (5 MINUTES)

Either read the following statement or use your own words:
The main goal of this program is to develop the mindset of a healthy female athlete. This is attained by defining and pursuing a healthy body ideal for athletes, using nutrition as fueling for better performance and health instead of dieting/restrictive eating, and learning techniques to resist unrealistic societal standards of beauty.

Rules and Expectations. Leaders make sure the rules are understood by the individuals. If someone doesn't feel they can follow the rules, they may leave at any time without repercussions.

1. Confidential Setting—athletes, leaders, and anyone involved cannot discuss any personal information outside this group with other individuals. It is OK to discuss lessons learned—nutrition, positive body talk, etc. can be discussed (just no identity-revealing information of other group members).
2. Again, we will have some light homework. It is beneficial to do this and write it down if asked.
3. Athletes do NOT have to discuss anything beyond what they wish.
4. NO CELL PHONES—understand this is a serious topic and full attention is needed.
5. There will be questionnaires at the beginning and end. Athletes can choose to fill these out and compare scores at the beginning and end. (Leaders should know that athletes are allowed to participate even if they do not wish to fill out these questionnaires.)

Leaders, please get a verbal agreement from each girl to abide by these guidelines.

If your program wants to use questionnaires, please hand them out and have the athletes fill them out. Either the athletes can keep the forms or the leaders can keep them until the end. It is up to each program.

DEFINING/DISCUSSING HEALTHY MINDSET AND BODY IMAGE FOR ATHLETES (20 MINUTES)

Leaders—Transition: To start this program, we are going to discuss what a healthy mindset and body image in sport looks like and how that can look different from the societal and social pressures we receive.

Discussion Questions

Who decides what an attractive female body looks like?

*   *Societal norms?*
*   *Adults?*
*   *Males? Females?*
*   *Figures in sports magazines, advertising, television, etc.?*

What is society's idea of an "attractive female body"? (Record these on a white-board/large notepad.) Pick an athlete to write.

- *Skinny but curvy in the "right" places*
- *Lean but not too muscular*
- *Thin, tall legs*
- *Tan*
- *Small nose and pronounced cheekbones*
- *Clear skin*
- *Straight, super white teeth*
- *Pretty eyes*
- *Looks "good" in a bikini*

What things in society perpetuate this myth of an attractive body?

- *TV (representation of only certain body types as "attractive" characters on TV or movies)*
- *Social media (fitness influencers, products from certain celebrities, photo editing)*
- *Advertisements (diet ads, products guaranteeing their product can give you "perfect" skin, hair, teeth, etc., unrealistic clothing ads)*

How often are these images touched up or photoshopped? Why is this a problem?

- *Very often—So often that there are bills being put forth to make sure photo-shopped images are labeled*
- *Gives a skewed perception of what "normal" bodies look like—Normal bodies have rolls, cellulite, crooked teeth, acne, and overall are imperfect— this image is not represented in edited photos*

What characteristics of the "attractive female body" are similar to perceptions of how athletes in your sport are told they should look (*answers will vary by sport*)? What does the perfect body look like for your sport?

- *Thin or muscular dependent on sport*
- *Lean/defined muscle tone*
- *Swimmer (strong arms and broad shoulders)*
- *Distance runner (super skinny with lean muscle)*
- *Sprinter (strong legs with an overall toned body)*
- *Basketball/Volleyball (strong arms, tall)*
- *Poms/cheer (blonde, long hair, looks good in a short skirt)*
- *Looks good in a swimsuit/uniform/etc.*

Leaders: There will be different definitions for each type of athlete, please focus on the sports present in your group.

Is it healthy for females to work towards having either of these body types?

- *No, these are unrealistic*

Why is it unhealthy to pursue a societally based "attractive female body"? Why is it also unhealthy to pursue the body type/image supposedly needed for your sport?

- *Both are unrealistic and promote a single body type (they lack an appreciation for body diversity)*
- *"Attractive female body"—Individuals may internalize unrealistic expectations of how they must look, heightening risk of disordered eating, overexercise, body dissatisfaction, and purchase of products falsely promoting obtainment of the "attractive female body"*
- *Sport body type/image—athletes may feel pressure to restrict their diet, overtrain or engage in other unbalanced eating/exercise habits to obtain the body type they believe is necessary to excel in their sport*

What attributes make a female athlete healthy?

- *Healthy functioning body (having good energy levels, having your period, lack of injuries)*
- *Nutrition balanced*
- *Appropriate sleep*
- *Fueling appropriately*
- *Mental wellness*
- *Healthy self-esteem*
- *Emotional and social wellness*

How does society expect females to behave in comparison to males? (Answers may vary depending on upbringing, cultures, religion, etc.)

- *Less strong*
- *Less tough*
- *Less risk-taking*
- *Less independent*
- *Less intelligent*
- *Less confident*
- *Less leadership*

Are these fair expectations? How are these perceptions detrimental to individuals in sports?

- *No—They are unfair to all genders and set dangerous stereotypes of how people must behave based on the outward appearance of sexual identity*
- *Limits opportunities for girls'/women's sports to be featured on television/media as it is not as "exciting" as boys'/men's sports*

- *Shames boys/men in sport for being vulnerable—They are not "manly" enough*
- *Strong girls/women are told they are "too masculine"*
- *Especially unfair to those who are transgender athletes or identify as gender fluid or nonbinary*

How does an athlete with a healthy mindset and body image look PHYSICALLY in comparison to the unrealistic expectations discussed? (Record these on a whiteboard.)

Examples

- *Possibly more muscular or less if they are new to the sport*
- *Likely a higher (and healthier) body fat percentage*
- *Different heights (not as tall or short as the ideal)*
- *Smaller or larger breasts*
- *No one prototype—everyone is different*
  ***Perhaps the most important take-home point

How does an athlete with a healthy mindset and body image look MENTALLY and EMOTIONALLY in comparison to the unrealistic expectations discussed?

- *Views food as fuel for training and performance*
- *Is not scared of eating food and healthy weight gain*
- *Feels okay treating themselves to "unhealthy" foods that they enjoy*
- *Has a positive image of muscle tone and is proud to be strong OR of not having as much muscle volume as others—Body confidence*
- *Has a positive image of her body in attaining goals (for swimming, running, basketball, general physical activity, etc.)*
- *Goals and nutrition are related to performance, improvement, and health rather than to the appearance of one's body*
- *Flexibility of mind to know that her body is not an indicator of who she is on the inside or of self-value*
- *Views athletes as all different sizes and shapes—Knowing that ALL body types can excel in their sport*
- *Positive self-esteem*

What actions can athletes take to achieve their goals of aiming to have a healthy mindset and body image? Include psychological, emotional, and mental factors.

Examples

- *Steady attendance at practice*
- *Take pride in hard sets/workouts—Even when they are tough*
- *Embrace all athletes as part of the team regardless of body type or other factors*
- *Eat nutrient-rich foods and make sure you are getting enough calories*
- *Prevent and take care of injuries (including not training through injuries)*
- *Lift weights and do strength work as appropriate*

- *Get adequate sleep*
- *Encourage teammates to view other female bodies in a positive manner*
- *Promote a culture accepting of every body type*
- *Recognize the difference between training hard and overexercising*

Who are some positive role model athletes who have a healthy attitude and prioritize their health and well-being over society's unrealistic ideals? What can we learn from them?

Varied answers

- *Simone Biles valued mental health at the Tokyo Olympics*
- *Serena Williams speaking out against stereotypical body types*
- *Norwegian beach handball wearing shorts instead of bikinis and being fined, but desiring practicality and modesty*
- *Paralympian runner Olivia Breen being ridiculed for wearing buns (tight small running shorts) and told it is too revealing, but competing in them as she feels more comfortable*
- *Germany gymnastics team chose unitards at the Tokyo Olympics as they felt more comfortable*
- *Naomi Osaka, Japanese tennis star who pulled out of the French Open due to mental health*

NUTRITION FOR THE SEASON (15 MINUTES)

Transition: Now, we will discuss how to use food to fuel your body for improved athletic performance and general well-being.

Discussion Questions (Leaders, please write answers on whiteboards/notepads.)

Why should we care about nutrition?

- *Nutrition as fuel for performance—Performance in sport, classes, and life in general*
- *Provides energy for sports performance, health, and life*
- *Allows us to build muscle*
- *Allows us to recover after meets/games/hard practices*
- *Eating right can prevent certain health issues (cardiovascular disease, type II diabetes)*
- *Carries social and cultural value—Enjoying holiday meals with family or post-competition milkshakes with the team is important, too*

What should we fuel with as female athletes?

- *Carbohydrates (pasta, bread, rice, quinoa, granola, etc.—aim for whole wheat or multigrain if possible)*
- *Fats (avocado, olive oil, coconut oil, etc.)*
- *Proteins (beef, chicken, pork, tofu, beans, fish, etc.)*

- *Veggies/Fruits (celery, broccoli, asparagus, apples, mangos, etc.)*
- *Vitamin/Minerals if we are not meeting certain needs in our diet (in particular calcium, vitamin D, and iron as female athletes)*
  - *Calcium and vitamin D = Crucial in building strong bones and preventing bone injuries in addition to premature osteoporosis*
  - *Iron = Necessary in helping our blood carry oxygen—low iron can be a common cause of fatigue in athletes especially female athletes who lose iron during their menstrual cycle*

Why is breakfast important?

Leaders: Discuss cortisol response when female athletes do not eat breakfast—cortisol is a hormone produced by our bodies when under stress. Leaders can share the associated "Importance of Breakfast" handout.

- *Our baseline cortisol is highest in the mornings. When we eat breakfast the cortisol levels go down. Skipping breakfast makes our bodies think we are in stress mode. When our body is in this perceived stress mode, we have a harder time regulating sugar levels, balancing metabolism, and fighting infections.*
- *By eating protein and carbs at breakfast, athletes can provide energy for afternoon practices.*
- *Without breakfast, we can become tired by the afternoon, impacting our practices and performances.*

What barriers may prevent someone from eating breakfast and how can we overcome these barriers?

- *Not enough time → Eat on the go (peanut butter toast with banana slices), prepare breakfast the night before (overnight oats)*
- *Not hungry → Start small and work your way up, try breakfast smoothies that contain all major food groups, ask yourself if you are eating a large late-night snack that prevents you from eating breakfast the next morning*
- *Afraid of gaining weight → Gaining healthy weight is not a problem—it can also be muscle weight. Again, the cortisol response can be discussed*

Training plate activity—Give each girl a handout and explain the training plate ratios. They can draw appropriate examples. *Mention the increased ratio of carbohydrates (an athlete's main energy source) on high-intensity days. Higher-energy expenditure = higher need for carbohydrates.*

Next session, we will further elaborate on the importance of eating breakfast as well as other meals and snacks by discussing Relative Energy Deficiency in Sport (RED-S) which can be common in female athletes.

HOMEWORK (5 MINUTES)

Homework: Come up with one nutrition goal and one mindset goal for positive change to work on in between this session and our next. Write down five positive things about your body and mindset that help your performance.

CONCLUSION (10 MINUTES)

Does anyone want to say one last thing or compliment a teammate on a positive attribute they have seen in them?

Leaders: Please make sure it ends on a positive note. If nobody has anything to say, compliment the group on the positive things they have said in session.

SESSION 2

Supplies—whiteboard or paper easel, markers, nine coins, homework handout, RED-S handout

Potentially 3–4 weeks into the season

    I. Introduction (5 minutes)
    II. Positive and Negative Self-Talk (10 minutes)
    III. RED-S (10 minutes)
    IV. Nutrition for Mid-Part of Season (20 minutes)
    V. Sleep (10 minutes)
    VI. Homework: Find a private spot and read aloud the positive things you wrote to yourself from last time. Write a new nutrition goal, positive body image goal, and sleep goal.
    VII. Conclusion (5 minutes)

INTRODUCTION (5 MINUTES)

If using social media, also recommend following SPRING Forward social media accounts for more extensive information.

- Instagram: @spring_forward_girls
- Facebook: @springforwardgirls
- Website: springforwardgirls.com

Remind athletes of the confidentiality agreement.
Remind athletes of the no cell phones policy.

Ice Breaker: Ask if anyone wants to share an example of a teammate showing positivity since the last meeting—sticking to a goal, working hard at practice, taking initiative with fueling their body, talking about their body in a positive way, etc.

    Review of Session 1: Follow-up from last session's homework sharing only if they want to. (Write down five positive things about your body and mindset that help your performance.)

Sharing of goals—Made it or not? It's important to note that athletes can choose to share none, some, or all of the homework from the last session—there's no obligation to share completely.

If nobody wants to share, talk about how hard it is to make positive statements about yourself. Even if athletes are not able to discuss, please ask if this task was difficult to do and why we find it so difficult to compliment ourselves. This will lead into the next segment.

Positive and Negative Self-Talk (10 Minutes)

Leaders—Transition: Now that we have just talked about how difficult it can be to make positive statements about ourselves, we want to turn our discussion to positive and negative self-talk.

Discussion Questions

What kinds of thoughts go through your head after a bad competition/workout? (Record these on a whiteboard/notepad.)

- *Disappointment in self (I suck at my sport; I should just quit; I will never get better and reach my goals)*
- *Self-doubt in personal capabilities (I am not fast; I just don't have a runner/swimmer/athletic build; I have bad genetics)*
- *Angry for not doing as well as teammates (I don't know why I am not as fast as my teammates if we do the same workouts)*
- *Guilt (I let my coaches, parents, teammates down; If I hadn't ate X I would have competed better; If I had slept X amount of hours, I would have competed better)*
- *Wanting to make changes to improve (Next time, I will warm up more; Next time, I will eat this before)*

How can we alter the negativity in these thoughts to be more positive and help us the next time we compete? (Leaders, use the thoughts recorded on the whiteboard.)

- *Disappointment in self → This performance was not what I wanted, but it does not define me. I can learn and do better next time.*
- *Self-doubt in personal capabilities → One bad race/competition does not make me a bad athlete. Improvement means learning from bad workouts/races.*
- *Anger at not doing as well as teammates → Each person has good and bad workout days. I am allowed to be disappointed, but I can still support and be happy for my teammates.*
- *Guilt → I compete in the sport for myself—my coaches, parents, and teammates' opinions regarding my performance do not invalidate my worth.*
- *Wanting to make changes to improve next time → Evaluate why my performance was not what I wanted and how I can improve.*

How can I utilize a bad competition/workout to make myself a better athlete?

Leaders: Please emphasize that athletes should not be afraid of failure and that negative self-talk is not needed. It is okay to be upset with a performance and use the experience to learn. Leaders use the whiteboard.

- *Changing nutrition to maximize fueling (this likely means eating more calorie-dense, nutritious food; getting three balanced meals a day; ensuring you are not at a caloric deficit)*
- *Working smarter (learning the needs of your individual body; finding the balance between undertraining and overtraining; maximizing performance in a manner that puts less wear and tear on your body;, being intentional with practices)*
- *Adding core/weights (trying to focus on being generally strong—emphasizing* strong *makes you compete better rather than being undernourished to fit a certain body type)*
- *Coming to practice more (consistency is key to improvement with sports)*
- *Commitment to good sleep (awareness of recovery and sleep in improving performance)*
- *Trying mental imagery (writing out an ideal competition, WIN (what's important now) acronym)*
- *Being receptive to advice from other athletes and coaches (being coachable is important to excel in sports—also recognize that you get to decide what advice you choose to take or not take)*

What kinds of thoughts go through your head after a great competition/workout?

- *I am a good athlete (I am fast; I was able to compete with people I normally cannot)*
- *I can accomplish my goals (I finally hit the time I wanted; I can go after an even faster goal)*
- *My work paid off (I am training right; I am fueling right; Getting more sleep is helping)*
- *Maybe still doubt (How did that happen; I just got lucky; Everyone else just had an off day; I could have done better)*

How can I utilize a good competition/workout to make myself a better athlete? (Leaders use the thoughts recorded on the whiteboard.)

- *I am a good athlete → Use these workouts to build confidence and remember them during moments of self-doubt*
- *I can accomplish my goals → Understanding you are capable*
- *My work paid off → Working diligently, eating healthy, training smart, and recovering can pay off*
- *Maybe there is still doubt → You performed the way you did because of YOU—if you do it once you can do it again; emphasize changing this negative self-talk to positive ways to build confidence*

NOTE to Leaders: It is important to still practice humility and support other teammates.

How does a bad competition/workout affect your perception of yourself and body image?

- *Ruins confidence (I am not a good athlete; I cannot hit my goal time; I just don't compete or work out well)*
- *Discouraged (I will never make the team I want; My hard work never pays off; I should give up)*
- *Poor body image (My legs, stomach, etc. is/are too big to compete at the level I want; I don't have an "athletic" body type; I am fat; I am not fit— even if you are fit at this time)*

How does a good competition/workout affect your perception of yourself and body image?

- *Confidence (I am a good athlete; I am a hard worker; I am a team player)*
- *Encouraged (I can make the team I want; My hard work is effective; I can accomplish my goals)*
- *Positive body image (I am so fit and strong; My body helps me accomplish the goals I want; I am proud of the way my body looks)*

Do you believe the way we perform in practice or competitions can alter the way we view our self-perception and body image?

- *Yes*

Do you think it is easier for us to use negative self-talk and beat up on ourselves rather than using positive self-talk to build ourselves up?

- *Yes*
- *Reference the homework from last time and difficulty complimenting ourselves*

So, why is it important we change negative self-talk to positive self-talk?

- *To build confidence both in our sport and outside our sport*
- *To make sure we do not limit ourselves in sports and outside sports*
- *To build a positive perception of ourselves both physically (body image) and in our capabilities*

How can negative self-talk apply to nutrition and our body image? And why do you think this negative self-talk can affect food and body image?

- *Feeling guilty for eating something unhealthy*
- *Guilt or fear over getting too "fat" for your sport*
- *Guilt of eating something that will hurt your athletic performance*

Leaders: Talk about some of the foods you eat that are not considered convention- ally healthy. Then talk about some of the conventionally healthy things you do eat. Encourage the girls to also share both their unhealthy and healthy nutrition choices.

Healthy foods are the key to fueling well for our season, but they can be taken to the extreme. If we restrict our eating we can cause our bodies to be deprived of the energy needed to improve performance. How can you balance eating healthy with ensuring you are not restricting your nutrition or depriving yourself of your favorite foods?

- *Making sure to enjoy one treat a day (eating a piece of chocolate each night; having my favorite treat alongside a healthy meal)*
- *Having a milkshake with a healthy meal after a race; eating a healthy recovery snack and having a treat*
- *Knowing it is okay to not have perfect nutrition and it is a goal to work toward balanced and sustainable nutrition (sometimes you will have to be flexible with what you are eating and that is okay!)*
- *Recognizing that food has cultural and social context as well—enjoying holiday meals, ice cream with friends or post-competition shakes with team-mates is also part of healthy eating; eating should be balanced*

Relative Energy Deficiency (10 Minutes)

Leaders—Transition: To continue our discussion of nutrition, we want to talk about why it is so important that you, as athletes, ensure you are eating enough healthy calories to fuel yourselves for sport.

Discussion Questions

What do you feel like when you haven't eaten for a long time—when you feel "hangry"?

- *Irritable/crabby*
- *Tired/sleepy*
- *Weak/lacking energy*

What do you think would happen if you didn't eat enough over several days?

- *Tired/sleepy*
- *Weak/lacking energy*
- *Difficulty focusing in school or practice*
- *Difficulty remembering information*
- *Body breaks down muscle and bone for energy*

Do female athletes typically get enough calories?

Female athletes frequently underfuel in comparison to their athletic needs. Under-fueling can lead to long-term issues in both athletics and your general health. This condition of underfueling is known as Relative Energy Deficiency in Sport (RED-S). We are going to go over a handout discussing the symptoms of RED-S and how we can avoid the development of RED-S.

RED-S Handout—Discussion Points

- *RED-S is multifactorial*
- *RED-S can lead to different outcomes in each athlete*
- *The severity of RED-S can vary widely*
- *Many aspects of RED-S can be reversed if dealt with early on*
- *Lifelong issues from RED-S can include fertility problems, poor bone density, and mental health issues (e.g. eating disorders, anxiety, depression)*
- *Bone density issues can be seen in teenagers (e.g. stress fractures and premature osteoporosis)*

NUTRITION FOR MIDDLE OF THE SEASON (20 MINUTES)

Leaders—Transition: To avoid the development of RED-S, it is important we ensure we are eating healthy as well as eating enough. We are going to go over some ways to properly fuel ourselves for practice and competition.

Discussion Questions

What should I eat before practice? And when should I try to eat before practice?

- *Carbohydrates and a little protein*
- *Snacks (banana or apple slices with peanut butter, protein balls, applesauce, dried fruit, trail mix, granola bar). If less than 45 minutes prior to practice, something more liquid with carbohydrates. If more than 60–90 minutes before practice, something low fiber, low fat, and easy to digest. Granola, protein balls, or high-fat nut butter are less helpful this close to practice time. They are more appropriate 2–4 hours out, especially for prone sports (swimming)*
- *Breakfast (bagel with peanut butter, oatmeal with fruit and peanut butter, peanut butter toast, Greek yogurt with an English muffin)*
- *Lunch (ham sandwich with apple slices, turkey wrap with veggies, chicken, and rice with cooked veggies)*
- *Dinner (chicken and rice burrito with salsa, spaghetti with meatballs, soup with a dinner roll)*

What should I eat to recover after practice?

- *Carbohydrates and protein as well as fluids*
- *Carbohydrates → Replenish energy stores depleted during exercise to quicken recovery and make sure you have sufficient energy for your next workout/competition*
- *Protein → Provides building blocks for muscle repair/growth*
- *Fluids → Replenish fluids lost in sweat during exercise*
- *Breakfast (eggs and toast/bagel, Greek yogurt and granola, pancakes with peanut butter or protein mix)*
- *Lunch/dinner (protein—chicken, pork, beef, tofu, beans; carbohydrates—rice, quinoa, bread, pasta)*

- *Snack (protein shake, chocolate milk, fruit with peanut butter or cheese sticks, celery, and peanut butter)*
- *Fluids (water, Gatorade, Nuun hydration tablets)—Can discuss tonicity of fluids if time. Electrolyte replacement? How long of exercise and how intense to need replacement? Under 1 hour this is likely not needed as water is enough*

What should I eat before meets and during meets if my events are far apart?

- *Carbohydrates and fluids*
- *Carbohydrates (granola bars, protein balls, granola, fruit, and veggies)*
- *Fluids (water, Gatorade, Nuun hydration tablets)*

What is the appropriate fluid intake for female athletes?

- *Water, electrolytes*
- *Soups*
- *Juices*
- *Watery fruits like watermelon, grapefruit, oranges*

Talk about monitoring urine color—Light lemonade is the goal color to look for.

Sleep (10 Minutes)

Transition: In addition to proper nutrition, sleep acts as a critical component of recovery.

Sleep Activity

Leaders: For this activity you will need nine coins (they can be any type as long as they are the same); the idea is that each hour of sleep you get is one coin and that each coin can then be "spent" on activities throughout the day; this activity is just meant to be a visual representation of how sleep allows us to do the activities we need throughout the day, emphasizing 8 to 9 hours of sleep/night for athletes.

Set up the coins and explain that each one is one hour of sleep. Ask the athletes what they spend these on during the day—this is a rough estimate.

Example—9 coins set out

- 3 go to hours of practice
- 5 go to classes
- 1 goes to time to eat

Example—Sleep-deprived 6 coins set out

- 5 go to classes
- What happens at practice and other times?

Discussion Questions

Why is getting enough sleep important?

- *To feel energetic*
- *To ease cravings for nutrient-poor foods and caffeine*

- *Help with school performance (feel focused for class next day, solidify memories from the day)*
- *Help with sport performance (recovery after workouts, critical time for muscle rebuild)*
- *Ease the risk of depression*
- *Hormonal balance*

What can I do to ensure I am getting 8 to 9 hours of sleep each night?

- *Time management throughout the day so not cramming at night*
- *Setting up a nighttime routine so easier to fall asleep*
- *Aiming to set a daily sleep schedule (go to bed and wake up at generally the same time)*

HOMEWORK (5 MINUTES)

- Find a private spot and read aloud the positive things you wrote to yourself last time.
- Write a new nutrition goal and positive body image goal as well as a sleep goal.

CONCLUSION (5 MINUTES)

Does anyone want to compliment someone on their efforts either during this session or in general?

Again—if nobody wants to talk, compliment the athletes for their efforts today and end on a positive note.

SESSION 3

Supplies—whiteboard or paper easel, markers, nutrition myths handout, carb-loading handout

   I. Introduction (5 minutes)
  II. Barriers to Goals (10 minutes)
 III. Nutrition for Competition (15 minutes)
  IV. What Have We Learned (15 minutes)
   V. Conclusion—Remember to hand out the "Post-Program Questionnaire and Feedback" (10 minutes)

INTRODUCTION (5 MINUTES)

Remind athletes of the confidentiality agreement.

Remind athletes of the no cell phones policy.

Ice Breaker: Ask if anyone wants to share an example of a teammate showing positivity recently or since the last meeting—sticking to a goal, working really hard in practice, taking initiative with fueling their body, talking about their body in a positive way, etc.

Review of Session 2: Follow up from homework last time—sharing only if they want (find a private spot and read aloud the positive things you wrote to yourself from last time; write a new nutrition goal and positive body image goal as well as a sleep goal).

Is it harder to read aloud the positive things about oneself than to think about them or write them down? Why do you think this is?

BARRIERS TO GOALS (10 MINUTES)

Transition: In order to have improved success reaching our goals—both the ones we did for the Session 2 homework as well as future goals—we are going to discuss different barriers/obstacles in goal-setting and how to overcome them.

Discussion Questions

What are the hardest parts of maintaining your nutrition goals? (Record these on a whiteboard.)

- *Feeling hungry or constantly thinking about food*
- *Desire to look thin*
- *Urge to have sugar or something unhealthy*
- *Unsure which foods to eat*
- *Hard to get the mindset of food as fuel for athletic performance*

What steps can you take in resolving each of these issues? (Use the thoughts recorded on the whiteboard.)

- *Feeling hungry or constantly thinking about food → This can be a sign of deprivation or underfueling with improper food groups, signaling a need to either eat more, eat more filling foods, or both*
- *Desire to look thin → We should remind ourselves that thin does not necessarily mean improved athletic ability; rather aim to feel healthy and strong*
- *Urge to have sugar or something unhealthy → Moderately treating yourself to your favorite foods is OKAY; restriction of these foods can lead to further craving and then binging*
- *Unsure which foods to eat → Reference information from our past session, our athlete handouts as well as our Instagram page (@spring_forward_girls), Facebook page (@springforwardgirls), or website (springforwardgirls.com) for more information pertaining to this*
- *Hard to get into the mindset of food as fuel for athletic performance → This is a process, so be forgiving with yourself and just try your best*

What are the barriers to maintaining a positive body image? (Record these on a whiteboard.)

- *Comparison to social media influencers or celebrities*
- *Comparison to other teammates or athletes*
- *Societal pressure to look a certain way*

- *Comments from other people about my weight*
- *I would just like to look thinner, curvier, have clearer skin, have straighter teeth, etc.*
- *My uniform make me self-conscious*
- *I am working on changing my body but not seeing the results I want*

What steps can you take in resolving each of these issues? (Use the thoughts recorded on the whiteboard.)

- *Comparison to social media influencers or celebrities → Disordered eating behaviors and poor body image are often perpetuated by these figures; images are fabricated; what you see is not necessarily healthy*
- *Comparison to other teammates or athletes → Each individual will have a different body shape and size that works for them*
- *Societal pressure to be skinny → Beauty does not mean skinny; beauty should be based on your character and how you make others feel*
- *Comments from other people about my weight → Only you determine how your body should look; coaches, teammates, friends, family, etc. do not have a say in this*
- *I would just like to look thinner → Remember this may not be best for your health; you should aim for whatever body will make you the healthiest*
- *My uniform makes me self-conscious → By aiming for a positive body image of yourself, perceptions of this may be decreased*
- *I am working on changing my body but not seeing the results I want → Ask if you are changing your body for healthy reasons; if you are changing your body for a healthy reason, are you doing so in the correct way (not cutting major food groups or restricting your diet)?*

What are the red flags for athletes and what should you do?

- *Someone being secretive about their eating*
- *Unexplained weight loss*
- *Loss of menstrual cycle*
- *Stress fractures*
- *Muscle cramping frequently*
- *Encourage healthy eating*
- *If severe, contact an adult—Coach, parents, guidance counselor, etc.*

NUTRITION FOR COMPETITION (15 MINUTES)

Transition: Now that we have discussed ways to combat barriers to healthy eating and positive body image, we are going to focus on nutrition for the big day—competition!

Handout—Nutrition Myths
What is a good pre-competition meal (e.g. dinner the night before a morning competition or lunch before an afternoon competition)? Encourage athletes to talk about what they would put on their plate and how much.

- *Make sure you have a plate with all food groups (protein, carbohydrates, veggies/fruits, fluids)*
- *Night before, aim for a larger meal if possible—Focus on carbohydrates to fuel competition the next day*
- *Right before the competition aim for something light and easily digestible if possible—Again focus on carbohydrates to provide quick fuel for competition*
- *NOTE: Each person will have different requirements before competition— test different meals during the season to know which help you feel and perform your best*

How should I fuel during my meet if I have multiple events or a long day of competition?

- *Carbs (granola bar, energy balls, pretzels, trail mix, etc.)*
- *Fluids (water, electrolytes, etc.)*
- *Timing of snacks—about 45 minutes before the event—May depend on the type of event. Similar snacks as prior to practice*

(This question is for endurance athletes who taper only.) How should an endurance athlete fuel during taper/end of season?

- *Eating a reasonable amount*
- *No need to make any significant dietary changes (keep some normalcy)*
- *Drink lots of fluids and try to stay hydrated*

What about specific needs?
It's important to understand that each person has different energy needs and so each person's nutrition will look different (do not feel ashamed if you need to eat more or eat different foods than your teammates, etc.)

- *Gluten-free*
- *Lactose issues*
- *Food allergies*

What are other issues that may occur with eating and athletics?

Leaders: Remind them that female athletes who have issues with amenorrhea or eating disorders may need additional help and they should seek resources to help if they feel at risk. DO NOT identify anyone as needing help in the group. If an athlete confides that they need help, discuss with director and parents and find resources best for their situation.

- *Not eating enough leads to amenorrhea or reduced energy*
- *Not timing meals/snacks correctly*
- *Eating foods that may aggravate your stomach before a competition*

What Have We Learned? (15 Minutes)

Transition: Now, we just want to have a brief overview of what we have learned from these past three sessions and what knowledge you have gained to make yourself a properly fueled and body-positive athlete.

Discussion Questions

What did you learn from this program that you did not know before?

Answers will vary

How can we as a team help to hold each other accountable for positive body talk and a healthy nutrition mindset?

- *Making positive compliments that are not centered on someone's body (saying "Wow you did so great at practice today—you are so strong right now" vs "You have been swimming so well—you look so skinny")*
- *Gently calling out teammates who make negative comments about others*
- *Reaching out to a teammate who looks like they are struggling*
- *Promoting healthy, non-restrictive eating habits at team meals*

What would you do if a teammate or friend was making a negative comment about eating or body image? (e.g. "This suit makes me look fat" or "Why are you eating that?")

- *Tell the teammate their comments are unwarranted and need to stop*
- *Remind the teammate that each person has different nutrition needs*
- *Remind the teammate that self-worth is not based on how your body looks*
- *If the issue continues, reach out to a trusted authority figure*

What would you do if you were on a team/club in the future and a coach was pressuring people to lose weight?

- *Find authority figures who are supportive of healthy eating/body image to speak with this coach*
- *Know how to seek help in a clinical setting (a physician, nutritionist, therapist, eating clinic, etc.)*
- *If you feel comfortable, approach the coach directly yourself and explain the issue with normalizing unhealthy eating patterns*

What would you tell younger athletes about nutrition and athletic body image? Especially those young athletes who look up to high school athletes?

- *Don't worry so much*
- *Remind them that bodies are meant to be different sizes and shapes*
- *Self-confidence should not depend on your weight*
- *You will perform better in sports if you are fueling properly rather than restricting*

What were your favorite takeaway messages from this?

Answers will vary

If your program wishes, hand out questionnaires and have the athletes fill these out if they wish. They can compare their answers to the beginning questionnaires.

CONCLUSION (10 MINUTES)

Either end by doing the positive comments activity as in previous session (athletes can randomly compliment teammates) OR preferably, try a positivity circle:

- One athlete sits in the middle and those surrounding say positive comments ranging from a time period of 30 seconds to 1 minute (depending on time restraints and group size). Have athletes take turns and ensure each person gets a chance to go who desires to participate.

9 Beyond High School
Info for Adult Women

Kathryn Vidlock
Rocky Vista University, Parker, CO, USA

Catherine Liggett
University of Colorado, Aurora, CO, USA

CONTENTS

WORDS TO KNOW

FERRITIN   A measure of iron stores.
FOLLICULAR PHASE   The follicular phase of the menstrual cycle starts on the first day of menstruation and ends with ovulation.
LUTEAL PHASE   The luteal phase of the menstrual cycle starts with ovulation and ends with the first day of menstruation.
RELATIVE ENERGY DEFICIENCY IN SPORT (RED-S)   A syndrome caused by energy deficiency, potentially impacting metabolism, hormones, menstrual function, bone health, immunity, protein synthesis, and heart function.

DOI: 10.1201/b23228-9

GENERAL INFORMATION

The prior chapters have explained the history and need for interventions for female athletes for both improving body image and nutritional knowledge. Female athletes of all ages can benefit from instruction in these areas, and there has been demand for this program to extend further. So, this section goes over information for collegiate and adult female athletes.

WHAT ARE SPRING AMBASSADOR ROLES AS ADULTS?

SPRING ambassadors are athletes who are peer leaders. As adults they will have more responsibilities than the high school ambassadors. They lead and facilitate the groups. They encourage and act as role models to their team and should have a strong desire to promote healthy nutrition for fueling and a mindset for positive body image. They are expected to read the background information, nutrition information, and RED-S information. More formal training may take place depending on the school. They are not expected to be experts. The leaders act as facilitators. They also may act as communication liaisons if an athlete is uncomfortable talking directly to an adult leader. If a SPRING Ambassador notices any red flags in an athlete, they should get a leader or the director involved immediately. They should not feel responsible for any diagnosis or treatment of RED-S or eating disorders. It is recommended to have one ambassador for roughly 10 athletes.

WHAT ARE THE GOALS OF EACH SESSION?

Session 1 goals focus on getting the group talking and feeling comfortable. The session starts off with an ice breaker. The basics of nutrition and the changes needed in nutrition over the season are discussed and the basics of body image and media influences.

Session 2 goals are furthering knowledge on nutrition. We discuss recovery nutrition and fueling appropriately for competition and sport-specific nutrition needs and discuss RED-S. We continue to discuss positive body image issues.

Session 3 goals are cementing the positive body image and empowering the female athletes to make good decisions as well as understand red flag behaviors in themselves and teammates.

One of the tools used is a positivity circle. One female athlete is in the middle and the others go around stating positive attributes of that athlete. Each athlete takes a turn in the middle. This may feel uncomfortable at first, but feedback is usually overwhelmingly positive.

PREVIOUS RESULTS

The SPRING Forward program has been used in schools in Colorado. The study used body image flexibility scores to assess change. Body image flexibility can be thought of as the "refers to the ability to openly experience thoughts or feelings about the body without acting on them or trying to change them.[1] The cross country/track team showed a statistically significant increase of 26.5% in body image flexibility. The cheer team showed an increase of 22.75%. Overall scores increased by 23.91%.[2]

WHAT ARE THE RED FLAGS A LEADER SHOULD WATCH FOR?

Group leaders, coaches, and parents should watch for red flags in female athletes. Behavioral changes include obsession with food, calories, and weight; avoidance of food-related activities; restrictive eating or binge eating; and frequent bathroom visits after meals. Physical changes may include excessive exercising, wearing baggy clothes, decreased weight or fluctuation in weight and body fat, stress fractures, hormonal abnormalities, loss of menstrual cycles, and increased growth of fine body hair. Psychological changes may include negativity about one's body, out of control feelings, and symptoms of depression and anxiety.[3] Most likely a leader will not have to deal with any of these, however, they should be prepared if it arises.

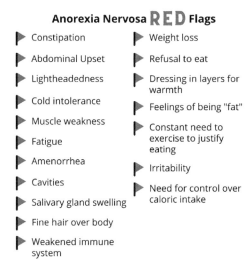

Anorexia Nervosa RED Flags

- Constipation
- Abdominal Upset
- Lightheadedness
- Cold intolerance
- Muscle weakness
- Fatigue
- Amenorrhea
- Cavities
- Salivary gland swelling
- Fine hair over body
- Weakened immune system

- Weight loss
- Refusal to eat
- Dressing in layers for warmth
- Feelings of being "fat"
- Constant need to exercise to justify eating
- Irritability
- Need for control over caloric intake

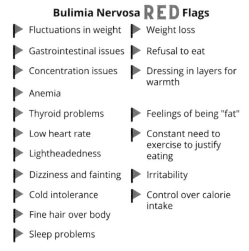

Bulimia Nervosa RED Flags

- Fluctuations in weight
- Gastrointestinal issues
- Concentration issues
- Anemia
- Thyroid problems
- Low heart rate
- Lightheadedness
- Dizziness and fainting
- Cold intolerance
- Fine hair over body
- Sleep problems

- Weight loss
- Refusal to eat
- Dressing in layers for warmth
- Feelings of being "fat"
- Constant need to exercise to justify eating
- Irritability
- Control over calorie intake

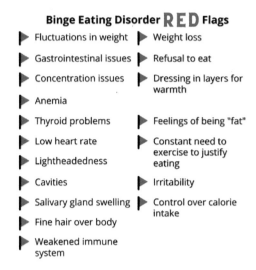

Binge Eating Disorder R E D Flags

- Fluctuations in weight
- Gastrointestinal issues
- Concentration issues
- Anemia
- Thyroid problems
- Low heart rate
- Lightheadedness
- Cavities
- Salivary gland swelling
- Fine hair over body
- Weakened immune system

- Weight loss
- Refusal to eat
- Dressing in layers for warmth
- Feelings of being "fat"
- Constant need to exercise to justify eating
- Irritability
- Control over calorie intake

Orthorexia R E D Flags

- Constantly checking food labels
- Concern over ingredients
- Cutting out food groups
- Unusual interest in what others are eating
- Showing stress when certain food options are not available

WHAT DO WE DO WHEN WE SEE RED FLAG SYMPTOMS?

It is recommended that every school have a plan in place for any athlete with red flag symptoms. This may be as simple as alerting a coach, athletic trainer, or athletic director. That responsible party will meet with the athlete. A plan to address the situation will be made, including possible intervention with physician, dietitian, psychologist, or another specialist. Always remember that confidentiality issues are of highest importance.

TROUBLESHOOTING

Missed sessions Our approach is to allow athletes to attend sessions even if they have missed a prior session. When possible, the group leader may choose to recap the previous session one on one with the participant.

Engagement At first the athletes may be hesitant to engage in the discussions. Usually, they will warm to the idea by the end of the first session. The hardest part for the athletes is often the friendship circle. They will likely enjoy complimenting other athletes but will have difficulty being in the center. It will help to maintain eye contact with the athletes. If needed, leaders can call on specific participants or go around the circle answering questions. If needed, remind them of the confidentiality within the group and encourage respectful remarks, especially if a participant is revealing personal issues.

Breaking confidentiality If a participant shares personal information outside of the group, the leaders should address the situation both with the individuals and the group. If serious enough the athlete may be asked to leave the program.

Homework There is a minimal amount of homework after sessions 1 and 2. We highly encourage the athletes to do the homework, but allow and encourage them to keep participating if they do not. The athletes who complete the homework generally feel they have learned more than those who do not.

Differences in knowledge, mindset, and sport abilities There will naturally be athletes of different levels. Our goal is to be inclusive and the information may be helpful to elite athletes as well as recreational athletes.

Let's discuss some of the concepts that are taught at the adult level.

FIRST AN OVERVIEW OF THE MENSTRUAL CYCLE

The follicular phase is from the first day of menstruation to ovulation. The first day of menstruation is when the cycle starts. The uterine lining falls away due to a lack of progesterone. During this phase, there is a low progesterone level and estrogen slowly rises to a peak. As ovulation occurs there is a peak in luteinizing hormone and an egg is released down the fallopian tube to the uterus.

After ovulation the luteal phase starts. The egg transforms into a corpus luteum and releases progesterone. If a sperm is not present, the corpus luteum withers and progesterone levels drop. Menstruation happens and the cycles continues.

DOES THE CYCLE IMPACT PERFORMANCE?

There is a lot to be learned about the effects of female hormones on performance. Unfortunately, many studies do not include females of childbearing age because of potential risks to a potential fetus. One study showed that performance is impaired during the midluteal phase of the cycle.[4] Another study showed that there may be slightly decreased aerobic capacity in the luteal phase, however this did not correlate to significant changes in overall performance.[5] There are studies looking at hydration status during the cycle, but again results are inconsistent.[6] Yet, we know that as little as 2% dehydration can cause impaired athletic performance.[7]

WHAT ABOUT NUTRITIONAL NEEDS DURING THE MENSTRUAL CYCLE?

Truthfully, this is an area where there are more questions than answers. It is known that progesterone increases the breakdown of protein while estrogen inhibits breaking down protein. So perhaps increasing protein during the luteal phase would be beneficial, but this is not fully studied.

Iron levels vary over the cycle and iron is lost with menses. Females are more likely to be diagnosed with iron deficiency or ferritin deficiency during menses.[8] It is also known that even if an athlete is not iron deficient to the point that she would be clinically diagnosed, she may benefit from increased iron for performance in distance running.[9] In addition, iron helps with recovery from both endurance and resistance exercise.[10] However, too much iron can cause toxicity, so anyone taking supplements should be under the care of a physician knowledgeable about iron and female athletes.

Athletes need to have calcium available for bone health. One component of RED-S is the lack of energy and the effect on bone density. Underfueling leads to decreased bone density and risk for stress fractures. In the United States the recommended intake of calcium for adults is 1000 mg a day. Is that enough for an athlete performing a sport that requires a lot of weight bearing? The answer is unknown. One study showed that consuming a pre-exercise meal of around 1300 mg calcium resulted in decreased markers of bone resorption, alluding to the fact that available calcium meant the calcium would not be taken from bone.[11] Another factor in bone metabolism and energy level is vitamin D. There has been controversy surrounding the level of vitamin D that causes insufficiency. One study proposes that athletes need higher levels, including over 50 nmol/L in winter or over 75 nmol/L in the summer.[12] It is known that long-term vitamin D deficiency may have negative cardiac effects.[13] Current recommended intake is 600 IU/day.[14] With the percentage of the general population and athletes that are vitamin D deficient, should this recommendation be raised? Again, athletes supplementing calcium or vitamin D should consult with a registered dietitian or physician familiar with the needs of athletes.

HOW CAN NUTRITION IMPACT PERFORMANCE?

So, understanding the above needs are important, but knowing what really affects performance is the real issue. Many studies are not performed during a specific time of the cycle.

A study on iron supplementation with 50 mg taken twice a day showed an increase in aerobic capacity and a decrease in energy expenditure. This was studied over the cycle and was found independent of the phase of the cycle.[15]

Vitamin D may also help performance. In a study of vertical jump ability, there was a substantial increase in the performance of athletes that took vitamin D 5000 IU daily.[16] Some studies have shown increases in strength and neuromuscular performance as well as decreased injuries. However, other studies have not repeated this finding.[17,18]

Caffeine is a known performance enhancer. Various studies over all phases of the cycle have shown increases in power and speed. However, too much caffeine can cause mood changes, jitteriness, and elevated heart rate.[19]

There are numerous studies on other supplements including cherry juice, beet juice, and various herbs. Currently, there isn't enough evidence to make a true recommendation.

TRAINING CONCEPTS

Many adult athletes using this program might be exercising on their own, while others may be part of a collegiate or professional team. Understanding the concepts of overreaching and overtraining are essential for peak performance. Functional overreaching is a normal part of training. An athlete lifts more, sprints more, or masters some aspect of training that is harder than the past. The athlete rests and comes back stronger. Nonfunctional overreaching is when the same aspect of training more or harder happens, but the athlete rests and there is no improvement. It may be too much. The athlete instead feels fatigued, and performance suffers. If this continues, overtraining happens. Overtraining can last for months, and an athlete may need significant time off. Some athletes have been driven to the point of quitting due to overtraining. Both nonfunctional overreaching and overtraining can take an emotional toll on an athlete.

AN ATHLETE'S STORY: Serina

I started dancing when I was five and started improving rapidly when I was 11–12. I moved to a more prestigious ballet academy and was competing against top-level girls in my area. The pressure was tremendous. My mom and I moved to a different city so I could advance. I did all my school online so I could dance many hours each day. My whole life was ballet. There was immense pressure to be as skinny as possible as that is thought to be more beautiful. Nobody talked about eating disorders, but most of the dancers restricted their eating to remain thin. This was thought to be normal. The perception of thin and fat was so different than normal. I knew that if I gained weight, I would have less chance to advance. I auditioned for many roles and companies and each time the girls who were some of the thinnest got the roles. I had instructors tell me I needed to lose weight. I had stopped getting my period at about age 17. I never thought twice about it being a medical problem. I was so hungry from the hours of practice, but I had to limit what I ate. I felt irritable and attributed it to the hard work.

Several years later, I auditioned to be a principal dancer and made it. This was a whole different world. If I thought things were bad before, they were certainly much worse now. I remember going out to eat with my family. I refused to go if I could not find a calorie count on the menu. I only ordered the low-calorie low-fat selections. I took nuts and cheese out of salads. I continued to be hungry all the time. My ballet friends said that my body would stop being so hungry after a while, but that never happened. I felt weaker and weaker and yet performed. I had numerous stress fractures over the years and problems with a tendon in my right foot. Still, I danced through.

I had an opportunity to audition for a more prestigious company. It was the obvious next step for my career. But my motivation was gone. I was tired of being weak and tired. I decided to stop ballet. My true friends and my family supported my decision. My family had been worried about me for some time, but they had not said much. They thought a ballet company would have given me appropriate nutrition advice. But we had no nutrition training, just comments made about being thin. I felt depressed after quitting and I started seeing a therapist. For the first time I learned about body positivity and saw the red flags that had happened for years. I fit all the categories of anorexia and had body dysmorphic disorder. I started medication for depression. I started gaining some weight.

It has been 10 years since I left ballet. I went to college and am now a financial planner. I don't want any further involvement with dance right now. I am afraid to go back to the mental state I once lived in. Many of the companies have nutritionists on staff now and I hope the changes are positive for those currently dancing.

CITATIONS

1. Linardon J, Anderson C, Messer M, Rodgers RF, Fuller-Tyszkiewicz M. Body Image Flexibility and Its Correlates: A Meta-Analysis. *Body Image*. (2021); 37: 188–203.
2. Vidlock, K, Liggett, C, Oberlag, N. Improvement of Body Image Flexibility in Adolescent Female Athletes Undergoing Education about Nutrition and Body Image. *Journal of Food Science and Nutrition Research* (2022); 5: 622–628.
3. Wells KR, Jeacocke NA, Appaneal R, et al. The Australian Institute of Sport (AIS) and National Eating Disorders Collaboration (NEDC) Position Statement on Disordered Eating in High Performance Sport. *Br J Sports Med*. (2020); 54: 1247–1258.
4. Freemas JA, Baranauskas MN, Constantini K, Constantini N, Greenshields JT, Mickleborough TD, Raglin JS, Schlader ZJ. Exercise Performance Is Impaired during the Mid-Luteal Phase of the Menstrual Cycle. *Med. Sci. Sports Exerc*. 2020; 3: 442–452. doi:10.1249/MSS.0000000000002464.
5. Lebrun CM, McKenzie DC, Prior JC, Taunton JE. Effects of Menstrual Cycle Phase on Athletic Performance. *Med. Sci. Sports Exerc*. 1995; 27: 437–444. doi: 10.1249/00005768-199503000-00022.
6. Giersch GEW, Charkoudian N, Stearns RL, Casa DJ. Fluid Balance and Hydration Considerations for Women: Review and Future Directions. *Sports Med*. 2020; 50(2): 253–261. doi:10.1007/s40279-019-01206-6.
7. Sawka MN, Burke LM, Eichner ER, Maughan RJ, Montain SJ, Stachenfeld NS. Exercise and Fluid Replacement. *Med. Sci. Sports Exerc*. 2007; 39: 377–390. doi: 10.1249/mss.0b013e31802ca597.
8. Kim I, Yetley EA, Calvo MS. Variations Menstrual during the Menstrual Cycle. *Am. J. Clin. Nutr*. 1993; 58: 705–709. doi: 10.1093/ajcn/58.5.705.

9. Woods A, Garvican-Lewis LA, Saunders PU, Lovell G, Hughes D, Fazakerley R, Anderson B, Gore CJ, Thompson KG. Four Weeks of IV Iron Supplementation Reduces Perceived Fatigue and Mood Disturbance in Distance Runners. *PLoS ONE.* 2014; 9. doi:10.1371/journal.pone.0108042.

10. Peinado A, Alfaro-Magallanes V, Romero-Parra N, Barba-Moreno L, Rael B, Maestre-Cascales C, Rojo-Tirado M, Castro E, Benito P, Ortega-Santos C, et al. Methodological Approach of the Iron and Muscular Damage: Female Metabolism and Menstrual Cycle during Exercise Project (IronFEMME Study) *Int. J. Environ. Res. Public Health.* 2021; 18: 735. doi: 10.3390/ijerph18020735.

11. Haakonssen EC, Ross ML, Knight EJ, Cato LE, Nana A, Wluka A, Cicuttini FM, Wang BH, Jenkins DG, Burke LM. The Effects of a Calcium-Rich Pre-Exercise Meal on Biomarkers of Calcium Homeostasis in Competitive Female Cyclists a Randomised Crossover Trial. *PLoS ONE.* 2015; 10: e0123302.

12. Wells KR, Jeacocke NA, Appaneal R, et al. The Australian Institute of Sport (AIS) and National Eating Disorders Collaboration (NEDC) Position Statement on Disordered Eating in High Performance Sport. *Br J Sports Med.* 2020; 54 (21): 1247–1258. doi:10.1136/bjsports-2019-101813.

13. de la Puente Yagüe M, Collado Yurrita L, Ciudad Cabañas MJ, Cuadrado Cenzual MA. Role of Vitamin D in Athletes and Their Performance: Current Concepts and New Trends. *Nutrients.* 2020; 12(2): 579. Published 2020 Feb 23. doi:10.3390/nu12020579.

14. Institute of Medicine, Food and Nutrition Board. *Dietary Reference Intakes for Calcium and Vitamin D*. Washington, DC: National Academy Press; 2010.

15. Dellavalle DM, Haas JD. Iron Supplementation Improves Energetic Efficiency in Iron-Depleted Female Rowers. *Med. Sci. Sports Exerc.* 2014; 46: 1204–1215.

16. Jones G. Pharmacokinetics of Vitamin D Toxicity. *Am. J. Clin. Nutr.* 2008; 88: 582S–586S. doi: 10.1093/ajcn/88.2.582S.

17. Bolland MJ, Grey A, Avenell A. Effects of Vitamin D Supplementation on Musculoskeletal Health. A Systematic Review, Meta-Analysis, and Trial Sequential Analysis. *Lancet Diabetes Endocrinol.* 2018; 6: 847–858.

18. Carlberg C, Haq A. The Concept of the Personal Vitamin D Reponse Index. *J. Steroid Biochem. Mol. Biol.* 2018; 175: 12–17. doi:10.1016/j.jsbmb.2016.12.011.

19. Helm MM, McGinnis GR, Basu A. Impact of Nutrition-Based Interventions on Athletic Performance during Menstrual Cycle Phases: A Review. *Int J Environ Res Public Health.* 2021; 18(12): 6294. Published 2021 Jun 10. doi:10.3390/ijerph18126294.

10 Session Manual for Adult Athletes

Kathryn Vidlock
Rocky Vista University, Parker, CO, USA

Catherine Liggett
University of Colorado School of Medicine, Aurora, CO, USA

Nicole Oberlag
Claremont College, Claremont, CA, USA

CONTENTS

DOI: 10.1201/b23228-10

SPRING AMBASSADORS

Before starting

1. Identify a mechanism of action for anyone who has red flag symptoms of an eating disorder. This could be as simple as alerting the athletic trainer at your school or a local physician or other health care professional who can help that athlete find resources.
2. Athletes should never feel pressured to answer anything they do not want. In that spirit, please do not call directly on any individual to answer in the group.
3. As a SPRING Forward Ambassador, please make sure to make every athlete feels included. We seek to include all athletes identifying as female, regardless of athletic level, body type, religion, race, or sexual orientation.

SESSION 1

Supplies—whiteboard or paper easel, markers, handout of homework, training plates, BI-AAQ Questionnaire

Timing: Early in the season

Topic Areas

I. Introduction (5 minutes)
II. Group Rules and Expectations (5 minutes)
III. Defining/Discussing Healthy Mindset and Body Image (20 minutes)
IV. Nutrition for the Season (15 minutes)
V. Homework—One nutrition goal and one mindset goal for positive change. Write down five things about your body and mindset that help your performance (5 minutes)
VI. Conclusion (10 minutes)

INTRODUCTION (5 MINUTES)

Leaders introduce themselves briefly. Take about 30 seconds.

- *What are your personal interests and passions?*
- *What are your past areas of study?*
- *What made you want to do this project?*
- *Did you struggle with these issues in the past or currently?*

Have the young women introduce themselves by saying their name and one thing they like about their body or mindset in approaching their health. (OK to use name tags if athletes do not know each other well.)

Remind participants that this program is educational and they may participate to the extent they desire including not participating at all.

There will be optional homework to do alongside attendance of three sessions. This homework is not required, but in exchange, athletes will hopefully benefit from improved nutrition, performance, and lifelong health benefits. They will likely get more out of this program if they complete the homework.

SPRING Forward social media—Recommend athletes navigate to the social media pages and follow if desired.

- Instagram—@spring_forward_girls
- Facebook—@springforwardgirls
- www.SPRINGforwardgirls.com

GROUP RULES AND EXPECTATIONS (5 MINUTES)

Either read the following statement or use your own words:
The main goal of this program is to develop the mindset of a healthy female athlete. This is attained by defining and pursuing a healthy body ideal for athletes, using nutrition as fuel for better performance and health.

Rules and Expectations. Leaders make sure the rules are understood by the individuals. If someone doesn't feel they can follow the rules, they may leave at any time without repercussions.

1. Confidential Setting—Athletes, leaders, and anyone involved cannot discuss any personal information outside this group with other individuals. It is OK to discuss lessons learned—nutrition, positive body talk, etc. (just no identity-revealing information of other group members).
2. Again, we will have some light homework. It is beneficial to do this, and write it down if asked.
3. Athletes do NOT have to discuss anything beyond what they wish. Athletes can be quiet the entire time or only participate in certain activities if they choose.
4. NO CELL PHONES—Understand this is a serious topic and full attention is needed.
5. There will be questionnaires at the beginning and end of the program. Athletes can choose to fill these out and compare scores at the beginning and end. (Leaders should know that athletes are allowed to participate even if they do not wish to fill out these questionnaires.)

Leaders: Please go around the room and get a verbal agreement from each athlete to abide by these guidelines.

Hand out the "BI-AAQ Questionnaires" and have them fill these out. The athletes can keep the forms or the leaders can keep them until the end. It is up to each program and athlete. If an athlete doesn't want to complete the questionnaire, that is fine.

DEFINING/DISCUSSING HEALTHY MINDSET AND BODY IMAGE (20 MINUTES)

Leaders—Transition: To start this program, we are going to discuss what a healthy mindset and body image in sport look like and how societally generated stereotypes are problems.

Discussion Questions

Who are some of the most famous and idolized female sports figures? (Record these on a whiteboard/large notepad.) Pick an athlete to write answers.

Examples: Answers will vary, especially by sport

- *Simone Biles*
- *Katie Ledecky*
- *Serena Williams*
- *Lindsay Vonn*
- *Alex Morgan*
- *Sue Bird*
- *Megan Rapinoe*
- *Kerri Walsh Jennings*
- *Mary Cain*

How have these athletes spoken out about body image?

- *Simone Biles—Valuing mental health at the Tokyo Olympics*
- *Serena Williams speaking out against stereotypical body types*
- *Norwegian beach handball wearing shorts instead of bikinis and being fined, but desiring practicality and modesty*
- *Paralympian runner Olivia Breen being ridiculed for wearing buns (tight, short running shorts) and told it is too revealing, but competing in them as she feels more comfortable*
- *German gymnastics team choosing unitards at the Tokyo Olympics as they felt more comfortable*
- *Naomi Osaka, Japanese tennis star who pulled out of the French Open due to mental health*
- *Mary Cain (track and field) speaking on coaching pressures related to body weight and running*

What is a body ideal?

- *A body ideal is a perception of how an individual's body should appear. This ideal may be held by society or a specific group.*

What does the perfect female body look like according to the general public?

- *Thin*
- *Large breasted*
- *Barbie doll–like figure*
- *Blonde*
- *Flawless skin*
- *White*

There are societal perceptions of how bodies should appear based on what sports athletes participate in. What are some examples? Answers will vary.

- *Cheerleaders should be skinny, tall, and large-breasted with blonde hair*
- *Runners should be thin and lean*
- *Softball players should look muscular*
- *Shot put athletes should be large*
- *Swimmers should be skinny but with strong shoulders*
- *Gymnasts need to be short and skinny*
- *Rowers need to have large shoulders*
- *Volleyball players should be tall with long arms and legs*

How does our perception of how athletes should look compare to society's perception of an ideal body? Think about differences in your specific sport.

- *More muscular dependent on sport*
- *Lean/defined muscle tone*
- *Flatter breasts*
- *Swimmer (strong arms and broad shoulders)*
- *Distance runner (thin with lean muscle)*
- *Sprinter (strong legs with an overall toned body)*
- *Basketball/Volleyball (strong arms, tall)*
- *Poms/cheer (blonde, long hair, looks good in a short skirt)*
- *Looks good in a swimsuit/uniform/etc.*

Leaders: There will be different definitions for each type of athlete, please focus on the sport(s) present in your group.

What types of things are done to perpetuate society's perception of a perfect female body?

- *Models are encouraged to starve themselves, many have disordered eating*
- *Performers are told they'll lose jobs if gain weight*
- *Already thin female bodies are photoshopped for the media*
- *TV and movies perpetuate the stereotype of stick-thin, large-breasted women as ideal*
- *Young girls are exposed to these stereotypes from an early age*
- *Girls feel pressured to attempt to attain a different body type by unhealthy means*
- *False information is often perpetuated on social media by "fitness influencers" who are not actually qualified to give health information*

As an athlete do you feel more pressure to try to obtain a perfect body type for your sport or one more like society's image?

Answers will vary

- *Many athletes feel some pressure to try to obtain both*
- *Many elite athletes care more about the ideal for their sport*

What happens when female athletes try to also achieve a stereotypical perfect body?

- *Super skinny bodies may not be sustainable for sport*
- *The athletic body may not align with societal ideals and may not be attainable for each body type*
- *Differences in body shape and size unique to each individual are ignored*
- *Health issues with trying to restrict eating and being energy deficient. These will be discussed later.*
- *Mental health—Frustration with trying to achieve something that is not healthy and not attainable without hurting oneself*

Not only are there body perceptions for athletes, but there are other societal perceptions that are not fair. What are examples (leaders may need to give an example to get started)?

- *Women bodybuilders look like men*
- *Softball players are all lesbians*
- *Cheerleaders and dancers are less intelligent*
- *The more muscle, the less the brain and vice versa*
- *Skinny runners all have eating disorders*
- *Athletic girls with short hair are LGBT*
- *Para athletes aren't real athletes*
- *Women's sports are less important than men's sports*
- *Women shouldn't be too muscular because they won't get a man*

How does an athlete with a healthy mindset and body image physically look in comparison to society's skewed expectations?

Examples

- *More muscular but potentially higher body fat percentage*
- *Different heights (not as tall or short as the ideal)*
- *No one prototype—Everybody is different. Perhaps the most important take-home point*
- *Someone new to the sport might not look as muscular as an athletic ideal*
- *All types are OKAY and aiming to look like the societal ideal can be unrealistic and dangerous*

How does an athlete with a healthy mindset and body image look mentally and psychologically?

Examples

- *Views food as fuel for training and performance in terms of her athleticism. Food may also be viewed as part of a religious or cultural role. For example, certain foods on holidays are entirely appropriate to eat*
- *Is not scared of eating food and healthy weight gain*
- *Feels okay occasionally treating themselves to unhealthy foods that they enjoy*

- *Has a positive image of muscle tone and is proud to be strong or not have as much muscle volume as others*
- *Has a positive image of her body in attaining goals (for swimming, running, general physical activity, etc.)*
- *Goals and nutrition are related to performance, improvement, and health rather than to the appearance of her body*

What actions can athletes take to achieve their goals of aiming to have a healthy mindset and body image? Include psychological, emotional, and mental factors.

Examples

- *Steady attendance at practice*
- *Take pride in hard sets/workouts—When they are tough*
- *Eat nutrient-rich foods and make sure you are getting enough calories*
- *Prevent and take care of injuries (including not training through injuries)*
- *Lift weights and do strength work*
- *Get adequate sleep*
- *Encourage teammates to view other female bodies in a positive manner*
- *Promote a culture accepting of every body type*
- *Watch negative body talk—Speak kindly to yourself*

Why is it important to develop a healthy mindset and body image as a female athlete?

Leaders: Write out the three different areas of benefit and examples.

Physical Benefits

- *Long-term health benefits*
- *Improved bone density*
- *Reduced rate of heart disease*
- *Better fertility later*
- *Fewer injuries*
- *Better performance*

Mental Benefits

- *Reduced likelihood of depression and anxiety*
- *Reduced likelihood of eating disorders*
- *Reduced likelihood of body dysmorphia*
- *More energy for school, work, sport, etc.*
- *Confidence*

Emotional Benefits

- *Better self-esteem*
- *Sense of personal empowerment*
- *Better engagement with peers—when you are happy with yourself, you will be able to better engage with others*

Nutrition for the Season (15 Minutes)

Transition: Now, we are going to discuss how to use food to fuel your body for both improved athletic performance and general well-being.

Discussion Questions (*Leaders:* Please write answers on whiteboards/notepads).

Why should we care about nutrition?

Examples

- *Nutrition as fuel for performance in sports, classes, and life in general*
- *Provides energy*
- *Our performance depends on it*
- *Allows us to build muscle*
- *Allows us to recover after meets/games/hard practices*
- *Eating right can prevent certain health issues (cardiovascular disease, type II diabetes)*

What should we fuel with, as female athletes?

Examples

- *Carbohydrates (pasta, bread, rice, quinoa, granola, etc.—aim for whole wheat or multigrain if possible)*
- *Fats (avocado, olive oil, coconut oil, etc.)*
- *Proteins (beef, chicken, pork, tofu, beans, fish, etc.)*
- *Veggies/Fruits (celery, broccoli, asparagus, apples, mangos, etc.)*
- *Vitamin/Minerals if we are not meeting certain needs in our diet (calcium, vitamin D, iron); it's important to note that the goal is to meet dietary requirements via our diet but female athletes can be prone to certain micro-nutrient deficiencies (particularly calcium, vitamin D, and iron)*

Why is breakfast important?

Leaders: Discuss cortisol response when female athletes do not eat breakfast—cortisol is a hormone produced by our bodies when under stress.

- *Our baseline cortisol is highest in the mornings. When we eat breakfast the cortisol levels go down. Skipping breakfast makes our bodies think we are in stress mode. The body has a harder time regulating sugar levels and metabolism and fighting infections*
- *By eating protein and carbs at breakfast, athletes can provide energy for afternoon practices*
- *Without breakfast, we can become tired by the afternoon, impacting our practices and performances*

What are barriers that may prevent someone from eating breakfast and how can we overcome these barriers?

Examples

- *Not enough time* → *Eat on the go, prepare breakfast the night before (over-night oats)*
- *Not hungry* → *Start small and work your way up, try breakfast smoothies that contain all major food groups, are you eating a large late-night snack that prevents you from eating breakfast?*
- *Afraid of gaining weight* → *Gaining weight is not a problem as it can be muscle weight. Again, cortisol response can be discussed*

Training plate activity—Give each athlete a handout and explain the training plate ratios. They can draw appropriate examples.

Carbohydrate—main energy source—on high-intensity days increase the ratio

Next session, we will further elaborate on the importance of eating breakfast as well as other meals and snacks by discussing Relative Energy Deficiency in Sport (RED-S) which can be common in female athletes.

HOMEWORK (5 MINUTES)

Homework: Come up with one nutrition goal and one mindset goal for positive change to work on in between this session and our next. Write down five positive things about your body and mindset that help your performance and/or your health.

CONCLUSION (10 MINUTES)

Does anyone want to say one last thing or compliment a teammate on a positive attribute they have seen in them?

Leaders: Please make sure it ends on a positive note. If nobody has anything to say, compliment the group on the positive things they have said in the session.

SESSION 2

Supplies—whiteboard or paper easel, markers, nine coins, handouts of homework, RED-S, and nutrition

Timing: Potentially 3–4 weeks into the season

    I. Introduction (5 minutes)
   II. Positive and Negative Self-Talk (10 minutes)
  III. RED-S (10 minutes)
  IV. Nutrition for Mid-Part of the Season (20 minutes)
   V. Sleep (10 minutes)
  VI. Homework: Find a private spot and read aloud the positive things you wrote to yourself last time. Write a new nutrition goal, positive body image goal, and sleep goal.
 VII. Conclusion (5 minutes)

Introduction (5 Minutes)

Remind athletes of the confidentiality agreement.
Remind athletes of the no cell phones policy.

Ice Breaker: Ask if anyone wants to share an example of a teammate or friend showing positivity recently or since the last meeting—sticking to a goal, working hard at practice, taking initiative with fueling their body, talking about their body in a positive way, etc.

Review of Session 1—Follow-up from last session's homework sharing only if they want. (Write down five positive things about your body and mindset that help your performance.)

Sharing of goals—Made it or not? It's important to note that athletes can choose to share none, some, or all of the homework from the last session; there is no obligation to share completely.

If nobody wants to share, talk about how hard it is to make positive statements about yourself. Even if athletes are able to discuss, please ask if this task was difficult to do and why we find it so difficult to compliment ourselves. This will lead to the next segment.

Positive and Negative Self-Talk (10 Minutes)

Leaders—Transition: Now that we have just talked about how difficult it can be to make positive statements about ourselves, we want to turn our discussion to positive and negative self-talk.

Discussion Questions

What kinds of thoughts go through your head after a bad race/workout? (Record these on a whiteboard/notepad.)

- *Disappointment in self (I suck at my sport; I should just quit; I will never get better and reach my goals)*
- *Self-doubt in personal capabilities (I am not fast; I just don't have a runner/swimmer/athletic build; I have bad genetics)*
- *Anger at myself for not doing as well as my teammates (I don't know why I am not as fast as my teammates if we do the same workouts)*
- *Guilt (I let my coaches, parents, and teammates down; if I hadn't eaten X I would have competed better; if I had slept X number of hours, I would have competed better)*
- *Want to make changes to improve (Next time, I will warm up more; next time, I will eat this before)*

How can we alter the negativity in these thoughts to be more positive and help us the next time we compete? (*Leaders:* Use the thoughts recorded on the whiteboard.)

- *Disappointment in self → This performance was not what I wanted, but it does not define me. I can learn and do better next time.*

- *Self-doubt in personal capabilities → One bad race/competition does not make me a bad athlete. Improvement means learning from bad workouts/races.*
- *Anger at not doing as well as teammates → Each person has good and bad workout days. I am allowed to be disappointed, but I can still support and be happy for my teammates.*
- *Guilt → I compete in sports for myself. My coaches', parents', and teammates' opinions regarding my performance do not invalidate my worth.*
- *Wanting to make changes to improve next time → Evaluating why my performance was not what I wanted and how I can improve.*

How can I utilize a bad workout/race to make myself a better athlete?

Leaders: Please emphasize that athletes should not be afraid of failure and that negative self-talk is not needed. It is okay to be upset with a performance and use the experience to learn. (Leaders use the whiteboard.)

- *Changing nutrition to maximize fueling (this likely means eating more calorie-dense, nutritious food; getting three balanced meals a day; ensuring you are not in a caloric deficit)*
- *Working smarter (learning the needs of your individual body; finding the balance between undertraining and overtraining; maximizing performance in a manner that puts less wear-and-tear on your body, being intentional with practices)*
- *Adding core/weights (trying to focus on being generally strong— Emphasizing strong makes you faster rather than skinny)*
- *Coming to practice more*
- *Commitment to good sleep (awareness of recovery and sleep in improving performance)*
- *Trying mental imagery (writing out an ideal competition, WIN (what's important now) acronym)*
- *Being receptive to advice coming from better athletes and coaches*

What kinds of thoughts go through your head after a great race/workout?

- *I am a good athlete (I am fast; I was able to compete with people I normally cannot)*
- *I can accomplish my goals (I finally hit the time I wanted; I can go after an even faster goal)*
- *My work paid off (I am training right; I am fueling right; getting more sleep is helping)*
- *Maybe still doubt (how did that happen; I just got lucky; everyone else just had an off day; I could have done better)*

How can I utilize a good workout/game/meet to make myself a better athlete? (Leaders use the thoughts recorded on the whiteboard.)

- *I am a good athlete → Use these workouts to build confidence and remember them during moments of self-doubt*
- *I can accomplish my goals → Understanding you are capable*
- *My work paid off → Working diligently, eating healthy, training smart, and recovering can pay off*
- *Maybe there is still doubt → You performed the way you did because of YOU—if you do it once you can do it again; emphasize changing this negative self-talk to positive ways to build confidence*

NOTE to Leaders: Important to still practice humility and support other teammates.

How does a bad game/meet/workout affect your perception of yourself and body image?

- *Ruins confidence (I am not a good athlete; I cannot hit my goal time; I just don't race or work out well)*
- *Discouraged (I will never make the team I want; my hard work never pays off; I should give up)*
- *Poor body image (my legs, stomach, etc. is/are too big to compete at the level I want; I don't have an "athletic" body type; I am fat; I am not fit— even if you are fit at this time)*

How does a good race/workout affect your perception of yourself and body image?

- *Confidence (I am a good athlete; I am a hard worker; I am a team player)*
- *Encouraged (I can make the team I want; my hard work is effective; I can accomplish my goals)*
- *Positive body image (I am so fit and strong; my body helps me accomplish the goals I want; I am proud of the way my body looks)*

Do you believe the way we perform in practice or competitions can alter the way we view our self-perception and body image?

- *Yes*

Do you think it is easier for us to use negative self-talk and beat up on ourselves rather than using positive self-talk to build ourselves up?

- *Yes*
- *Reference the homework from last time and difficulty complimenting ourselves*

So, why is it important we change negative self-talk to positive self-talk?

- *To build confidence both in our sport and outside our sport*
- *To make sure we do not limit ourselves in sports and outside sports*
- *To build a positive perception of ourselves both physically (body image) and in our capabilities*

How can negative self-talk apply to nutrition and our body image? And why do you think this negative self-talk can affect food and body image?

- *Feeling guilty for eating something unhealthy*
- *Guilt or fear over getting too "fat" for your sport or being different than the ideal body*
- *The guilt of eating something that will hurt your athletic performance*

Leaders: Talk about some of the foods you eat that are not healthy. Then talk about some of the healthy things you do eat. Encourage the women to also share both their unhealthy and healthy nutrition choices.

Healthy foods are the key to fueling well for our season, but they can be taken to the extreme. If we restrict our eating we can cause our bodies to be deprived of the energy needed to improve performance. How can you balance eating healthy with ensuring you are not restricting your nutrition or depriving yourself of your favorite foods?

Examples

- *Giving myself a treat when I am craving one (eating a piece of chocolate each night; having my favorite treat alongside a healthy meal)*
- *Knowing it is okay to not have perfect nutrition and it is a goal to work toward balanced and sustainable nutrition (sometimes you will have to be flexible with what you are eating and that is okay!)*

RELATIVE ENERGY DEFICIENCY (10 MINUTES)

Leaders—Transition: To continue our discussion of nutrition, we want to talk about why it is so important that you, as athletes, ensure you are eating enough healthy calories to fuel yourselves for sport.

Discussion Questions

What do you feel like when you haven't eaten for a long time—when you feel "hangry"?

- *Irritable/crabby*
- *Tired/sleepy*
- *Weak/lacking energy*

What do you think would happen if you didn't eat enough over several days?

- *Tired/sleepy*
- *Weak/lacking energy*
- *Difficulty focusing in school or practice*
- *Difficulty remembering information*
- *Body—break down of muscle and bone*

Do female athletes typically get enough calories?

- *Female athletes can frequently underfuel in comparison to their athletic needs. Underfueling can lead to long-term issues in both athletics and your general health. This condition of underfueling is known as reduced energy deficiency in sport (RED-S). We are going to go over a handout discussing the symptoms of RED-S, and how we can avoid the development of RED-S.*

RED-S Handout—Discussion Points

- *RED-S is multifactorial*
- *RED-S can lead to different outcomes in each athlete*
- *The severity of RED-S can vary widely*
- *Many aspects of RED-S can be reversed if dealt with early on*
- *Lifelong issues can include fertility problems, decreased bone density, and mental health issues*
- *Bone density issues can be seen even in teenagers*

NUTRITION FOR MIDDLE OF THE SEASON (20 MINUTES)

Leaders—Transition: To avoid the development of RED-S, it is important we ensure we are eating healthy as well as eating enough. We are going to go over some ways to properly fuel ourselves for practice and competition.

Handout—Nutrition Basics

Discussion Questions

What should I eat before practice? And when should I try to eat before practice?

- *Carbohydrates and maybe a little protein*
- *Snacks (banana or apple slices with peanut butter, protein balls, applesauce, dried fruit, trail mix, granola bar); if less than 45 minutes before practice, eat something more liquid with carbohydrates. If more than 60–90 minutes before practice, something low fiber, low fat, and easy to digest. Granola, protein balls, or high-fat nut butter may be less helpful this close to practice time. Foods high in fiber and fat can contribute to gastrointestinal distress for certain athletes if they are eaten too close to practice. They are more appropriate for 2–4 hours out, especially for prone sports (swimming).*
- *Breakfast (bagel with peanut butter, oatmeal with fruit and peanut butter, peanut butter toast, Greek yogurt with carbs) – even if the practice is early in the morning, it is still important to get a quick carbohydrate source in*

What should I eat to recover after practice?

Examples

- *Carbohydrates and protein; restore fluids lost in sweat*
- *Breakfast (eggs and toast/bagel, Greek yogurt and granola, pancakes with peanut butter or protein mix)*

- *Lunch/dinner (protein—chicken, pork, beef, tofu, beans; carbohydrates— rice, quinoa, bread, pasta)*
- *Snack (protein shake, chocolate milk, fruit with peanut butter or cheese sticks, celery, and peanut butter)*
- *Fluids (water, Gatorade, Nuun hydration tablets)—can discuss tonicity of fluids if time. Tonicity—These fluids all have less salt than your regular plasma (fluids in your bloodstream). So overuse of water and electrolyte products can lead to problems with overhydration.*
- *Electrolyte replacement? How long of exercise and how intense to need replacement? Under 1 hour this is likely not needed as water is enough.*

What should I eat before and during competitions if my events are far apart?

- *Carbohydrates and fluids*
- *Carbohydrates (granola bars, protein balls, granola, fruit, and veggies)*
- *Fluids (water, electrolyte drinks)*

What are different sources you can use to increase fluid intake? What is the appropriate fluid intake for female athletes?

- *Water, electrolyte drink*
- *Soups*
- *Juices*
- *Watery fruits like watermelon, grapefruit, oranges*
- *Talk about monitoring urine color—Light lemonade is a goal color to look for*

Sleep (10 Minutes)

Transition: In addition to proper nutrition, sleep acts as a critical component of recovery.

Discussion Questions

Why is getting enough sleep important?

- *To feel energetic*
- *To ease cravings and caffeine*
- *Help with school performance (feel focused for class the next day, solidify memories from the day)*
- *Help with sports performance (recovery after workouts, critical time for muscle rebuild)*
- *Ease the risk of depression*
- *Hormonal balance*

What can I do to ensure I am getting 8–9 hours of sleep each night?

- *Time management throughout the day so not cramming at night*
- *Setting up a nighttime routine so easier to fall asleep*
- *Aiming to set a daily sleep schedule (go to bed and wake up at generally the same time)*

HOMEWORK (5 MINUTES)

- Find a private spot and read aloud the positive things you wrote to yourself last time.
- Write a new nutrition goal and positive body image goal as well as a sleep goal.

CONCLUSION (5 MINUTES)

Does anyone want to compliment someone on their efforts either during this session or in general?

Again, if nobody wants to talk, compliment the athletes for their efforts today and end on a positive note.

SESSION 3

Supplies—whiteboard or paper easel, markers, handouts of nutrition myths, and carb-loading information

I. Introduction (5 minutes)
II. Barriers to Goals (10 minutes)
III. Healthy Exercise and the Menstrual Cycle (15 minutes)
IV. What Have We Learned (15 minutes)
V. Conclusion—Remember to hand out the "Post-Program Questionnaire and Feedback" (10 minutes)

INTRODUCTION (5 MINUTES)

Remind athletes of the confidentiality agreement.
Remind athletes of the no cell phones policy.

Ice Breaker: Ask if anyone wants to share an example of a teammate showing positivity recently or since the last meeting—sticking to a goal, working really hard in practice, taking initiative with fueling their body, talking about their body in a positive way, etc.

Review of Session 2: Follow-up from homework last time—sharing only if they want (*find a private spot and read aloud the positive things you wrote to yourself from last time*; *write a new nutrition goal and positive body image goal as well as a sleep goal*).

Is it harder to read aloud the positive things about oneself than to think about them or write them down? Why do you think this is?

BARRIERS TO GOALS (10 MINUTES)

Transition: In order to have improved success reaching our goals—both the ones we did for the Session 2 homework as well as future goals—we are going to discuss different barriers/obstacles in goal setting and how to overcome them.

Discussion Questions

What are the hardest parts of maintaining your nutrition goals? (Record these on a whiteboard.)

- *Feeling hungry or constantly thinking about food*
- *Desire to fit into an ideal body type*
- *Urge to have sugar or something unhealthy*
- *Unsure which foods to eat*
- *Hard to get the mindset of food as fuel for athletic performance*

What steps can you take in resolving each of these issues? (Use the thoughts recorded on the whiteboard.)

- *Feeling hungry or constantly thinking about food → This can be a sign of deprivation or underfueling with improper food groups, signaling a need to either eat more, eat more filling foods, or both*
- *Desire to fit into a body ideal → We should remind ourselves that unrealistic body ideals do not necessarily mean improved athletic ability; instead, aim to feel healthy and strong*
- *Urge to have sugar or something unhealthy → Moderately treating yourself to your favorite foods is OKAY; restriction of these foods can lead to further craving and then binging*
- *Unsure which foods to eat → Reference information from our past session, our athlete handouts, and our Instagram page (@spring_forward_girls), Facebook page (@springforwardgirls), and website (springforwardgirls. com) for more information about this*
- *Hard to get into the mindset of food as fuel for athletic performance → This is a process, so be forgiving with yourself and just try your best*

What are the barriers to maintaining a positive body image? (Record these on a whiteboard.)

- *Comparison to social media influencers or celebrities*
- *Comparison to other teammates or athletes*
- *Societal pressure to be skinny*
- *Comments from other people about my weight*
- *I would just like to look thinner/change a certain aspect of my body*
- *My uniform makes me self-conscious*
- *I am working on changing my body but not seeing the results I want*

What steps can you take in resolving each of these issues? (Use the thoughts recorded on the whiteboard.)

- *Comparison to social media influencers or celebrities → Disordered eating behaviors and poor body image are often perpetuated by these figures; images are fabricated; what you see is not necessarily healthy*
- *Comparison to other teammates or athletes → Each individual will have a different body shape and size that works for them*
- *Societal pressure to be skinny/change a certain aspect of my body → Beauty does not mean skinnier, more toned arms, or whatever other physical*

attribute you may feel pressure to achieve; beauty should be based on your character and how you make others feel
- *Comments from other people about my weight → Only you determine how your body should look; coaches, teammates, friends, family, etc. do not have a say in this*
- *I would just like to look thinner → Remember this may not be best for your health; you should aim for whatever body will make you the healthiest*
- *My uniform makes me self-conscious → By aiming for a positive body image of yourself, perceptions of this may be decreased*
- *I am working on changing my body but not seeing the results I want → Ask if you are changing your body for health reasons; if you are changing your body for a healthy reason, are you doing so in the correct way (not cutting major food groups or restricting your diet)?*

What are the red flags for athletes and what should you do?

- *Someone being secretive about their eating*
- *Unexplained weight loss*
- *Loss of menstrual cycle*
- *Stress fractures*
- *Muscle cramping frequently*
- *Encourage healthy eating*
- *If severe, contact an adult—Coach, parents, guidance counselor, etc.*

HEALTHY EXERCISE AND THE MENSTRUAL CYCLE (15 MINUTES)

Let's switch gears and talk about balanced exercise, overreaching, and overtraining.

Discussion Questions

What is overreaching? Overreaching can be thought of as two things.

- *Functional overreaching is a normal part of an athlete's season. This is adding new components of training, higher intensity, and faster sets, with results in better performance. Athletes have rest periods and improve.*
- *Nonfunctional overreaching happens when athletes practice faster, have intensity, lift bigger weights, and yet do not have improvements and in fact, may backslide.*

What is overtraining?

- *Overtraining may start as nonfunctional overreaching, but the decrease in performance lasts longer, potentially many months. There can be associated symptoms of fatigue, weakened immune systems, endocrine problems, and psychological issues. If not corrected, this can end an athlete's career.*

What does a healthy mental approach versus an unhealthy mental approach to exercise look like?

- A healthy athlete is eager to improve and enjoys being an athlete. They may get frustrated during a hard workout or have moments where it doesn't seem fun, but overall they are happy to be competing in their sport.
- A mentally unhealthy approach may be an athlete who has no desire to compete or practice. They may only continue to do so because of parental influence, the need for a scholarship, or other pressures.
- Another type of unhealthy approach may involve an athlete who is exercising to try to fit a body image type and allows eating certain foods dependent on their workout that day.

Let's talk about the cycle and how nutrition may affect that.
Why is it considered improper to talk about our cycles?

- *Women and girls have been taught to keep this private*
- *Some may have been taught that it would be embarrassing to speak about it*
- *Jokes made by society—"She must be on her period"*
- *Fear of being thought of as less because of symptoms*

What are the changes that we can notice as athletes during the cycle? Leaders may want to remind them that the cycle has four phases—menstrual, follicular (estrogen rises), ovulation, and luteal (progesterone rises)

- *Hungrier at times*
- *Mood changes—irritability*
- *Physical cramps*
- *Fatigue*

How does my cycle affect my performance?

- *There is some evidence that performance may be impaired during the mid-luteal phase (between ovulation and menses).*

Should I make nutrition changes during my cycle?

- *That is controversial as some studies show some gains but there is not enough evidence to know for sure.*

What changes might be helpful?

- *Eating when hungry*
- *Iron supplementation—May help with energy and endurance*
- *Calcium—May help with bone density*
- *Vitamin D—May help with energy and jumping power*
- *Protein increase—Progesterone-heavy phase (luteal) breaks down more protein*
- *Mango, beet, cherry juices—May be helpful, but little is known*

**Leaders: Please stress that any supplementation needs to be done with monitoring and consulting a physician and/or a dietitian.

What Have We Learned? (15 Minutes)

Transition: Now, we just want to have a brief overview of what we have learned from these past three sessions and what knowledge you have gained to make yourself a properly fueled and body-positive athlete.

Discussion Questions

What did you learn from this program that you did not know before?

Answers will vary

How can we as a team help to hold each other accountable for positive body talk and a healthy nutrition mindset?

- *Making positive compliments that are not centered on someone's body (saying "wow you did so great at practice today—you are so strong right now" vs. "you have been swimming so well—you look so skinny")*
- *Calling out teammates who make negative comments about others*
- *Reaching out to a teammate who looks like they are struggling*
- *Promoting healthy, non-restrictive eating habits at team meals*

What would you do if a teammate or friend was making a negative comment about eating or body image (e.g. "this suit makes me look fat" or "why are you eating that?")

- *Tell the teammate their comments are unwarranted and need to stop*
- *Remind the teammate that each person has different nutrition needs*
- *Remind the teammate that self-worth is not based on how your body looks*
- *If the issue continues, reach out to a trusted authority figure*

What would you do if you were on a team/club and a coach was pressuring people to lose weight?

- *Find authority figures who are supportive of healthy eating/body image to speak with this coach*
- *Know how to seek help in a clinical setting (a physician, nutritionist, therapist, eating clinic, etc.)*
- *If you feel comfortable, approach the coach directly and explain the issue with normalizing unhealthy eating patterns*

What would you tell younger athletes about nutrition and athletic body image? Especially those young athletes who look up to older athletes?

- *Don't worry so much*
- *Remind them that bodies are meant to be different sizes and shapes*
- *Self-confidence doesn't need to depend on your weight*

- *Restricting your eating under the impression it will make you compete better never works out—it leads to higher injury and increased risk of eating disorder*
- *Athletes of all bodies can be successful in their sport*
- *Other people don't get to decide how you look, eat, or exercise—you should always have a say in your body and health*

What were your favorite takeaway messages from this?

Answers will vary

Hand out body flexibility questionnaires and have the athletes fill these out if they wish. They can compare their answers to the beginning questionnaire.

CONCLUSION (10 MINUTES)

Either end by doing positive comments activity as in the previous session (athletes can randomly compliment teammates) OR preferably, try a positivity circle:

One athlete sits in the middle and those surrounding say positive comments ranging from the time period of 30 seconds to 1 minute (depending on time restraints and group size). Have athletes take turns and ensure each person gets a chance to go who desires to participate.

11 One-Time Session Manual

Kathryn Vidlock

Rocky Vista University, Parker, CO, USA

Catherine Liggett

University of Colorado School of Medicine, Aurora, CO, USA

CONTENTS

WORDS TO KNOW

RELATIVE ENERGY DEFICIENCY IN SPORT (RED-S) A syndrome caused by energy deficiency, potentially impacting metabolism, hormones, menstrual function, bone health, immunity, protein synthesis, and heart function.

INTRODUCTION

At times, there may be an opportunity to speak with female athletes in a more limited timeframe. This manual provides an outline for such times.

SESSION MANUAL

Supplies—whiteboard or paper easel, markers, homework handout, training plates handout, RED-S handout

DOI: 10.1201/b23228-11

Topic Areas

    I. Introduction and Group Rules and Expectations (5 minutes)
   II. Defining/Discussing Healthy Mindset and Body Image (20 minutes)
  III. Nutrition (15 minutes)
  IV. RED-S (10 minutes)
   V. Homework (5 minutes) * Optional
  VI. Conclusion (10 minutes)

INTRODUCTION AND GROUP RULES AND EXPECTATIONS (5 MINUTES)

Leaders introduce themselves briefly. Take about 30 seconds. Potential ideas:

What are your personal interests and passions?
What are your past areas of study?
What made you want to do this project?
Did you struggle with these issues as a high school athlete?

Have the girls introduce themselves—give their name and one thing they like about their body or mindset.

Remind participants that this program is educational, and they may participate to the extent they desire, including not participating at all.

If using social media, also recommend following SPRING Forward social media accounts for more extensive information.

- Instagram: @spring_forward_girls
- Facebook: @springforwardgirls
- Website: springforwardgirls.com

Either read the following statement or use your own words:
The main goal of this program is to develop the mindset of a healthy female athlete. This is attained by defining and pursuing a healthy body ideal for athletes, using nutrition as fuel for better performance and health instead of dieting/restrictive eating, and learning techniques to resist unrealistic societal standards of beauty.

Rules and Expectations. Leaders make sure the rules are understood by all individuals. If someone doesn't feel they can follow the rules, they may leave at any time without repercussions.

1. Confidential Setting—athletes, leaders, and anyone involved cannot discuss any personal information outside this group with other individuals. It is OK to discuss lessons learned—nutrition, positive body talk, etc. can be discussed (just no identity-revealing information of other group members)
2. Athletes do NOT have to discuss anything beyond what they wish.
3. NO CELL PHONES—understand this is a serious topic and full attention is needed.

Leaders: Please get a verbal agreement from each girl to abide by these guidelines.

**DEFINING/DISCUSSING HEALTHY MINDSET AND BODY IMAGE FOR ATHLETES
(20 MINUTES)**

Leaders—Transition: To start this program, we are going to discuss what a healthy mindset and body image in sport look like and how that can look different from the societal and social pressures we receive.

Discussion Questions

Who decides what an attractive female body looks like?

- *Societal norms?*
- *Adults?*
- *Males? Females?*
- *Figures in sports magazines, advertising, television, etc.?*

What is society's idea of an "attractive female body?" (Record these on a whiteboard/large notepad. Pick an athlete to write.)

- *Skinny but curvy in the "right" places*
- *Lean but not too muscular*
- *Thin, tall legs*
- *Tan*
- *Small nose and pronounced cheekbones*
- *Clear skin*
- *Straight, super white teeth*
- *Pretty eyes*
- *Looks "good" in a bikini*

What things in society perpetuate this myth of an attractive body?

- *TV (representation of only certain body types as "attractive" characters on TV or movies)*
- *Social media (fitness influencers, products from certain celebrities, photo editing)*
- *Advertisements (diet ads, products guaranteeing their product can give you "perfect" skin, hair, teeth, etc., unrealistic clothing ads)*

How often are these images touched up or photoshopped? Why is this a problem?

- *Very often—So often that there are bills being put forth to make sure photoshopped images are labeled*
- *Gives a skewed perception of what "normal" bodies look like—Normal bodies have rolls, cellulite, crooked teeth, acne, and overall are imperfect; this image is not represented in edited photos*

What characteristics of the "attractive female body" are similar to perceptions of how athletes in your sport are told they should look (*answers will vary by sport*)? What does the perfect body look like for your sport?

- *Thin or muscular, dependent on sport*
- *Lean/defined muscle tone*
- *Swimmer (strong arms and broad shoulders)*
- *Distance runner (super skinny with lean muscle)*
- *Sprinter (strong legs with an overall toned body)*
- *Basketball/Volleyball (strong arms, tall)*
- *Poms/cheer (blonde, long hair, looks good in a short skirt)*
- *Looks good in a swimsuit/uniform/etc.*

Leaders: There will be different definitions for each type of athlete—please focus on the sports present in your group.

Is it healthy for females to work toward having these body types?

- *No, these are unrealistic*

Why is it unhealthy to pursue a societally based "attractive female body"? Why is it also unhealthy to pursue the body type/image supposedly needed for your sport?

- *Both are unrealistic and promote a single body type (they lack an appreciation for body diversity)*
- *"Attractive female body"—Individuals may internalize unrealistic expectations of how they must look, heightening the risk of disordered eating, over-exercise, body dissatisfaction, and purchase of products falsely promoting obtainment of the "attractive female body"*
- *Sport body type/image—Athletes may feel pressure to restrict their diet, overtrain, or engage in other unbalanced eating/exercise habits to obtain the body type they believe is necessary to excel in their sport*

What attributes make a female athlete healthy?

- *Healthy functioning body (having good energy levels, having your period, lack of injuries)*
- *Nutrition balanced*
- *Appropriate sleep*
- *Fueling appropriately*
- *Mental wellness*
- *Healthy self-esteem*
- *Emotional and social wellness*

How does society expect females to behave in comparison to males? (answers may vary depending on upbringing, cultures, religion, etc.)

- *Less strong*
- *Less tough*
- *Less risk-taking*
- *Less independent*

- *Less intelligent*
- *Less confident*
- *Less leadership*

Are these fair expectations? How are these perceptions detrimental to individuals in sports?

- *No—They are unfair to all genders and set dangerous stereotypes of how people must behave based on the outward appearance of sexual identity*
- *Limits opportunities for girls'/women's sports to be featured on television/ media as it is not as "exciting" as boys'/men's sports*
- *Shames boys/men in sports for being vulnerable—They are not "manly" enough*
- *Strong girls/women are told they are "too masculine"*
- *Especially unfair to those who are transgender athletes or identify as gender fluid or nonbinary*

How does an athlete with a healthy mindset and body image look PHYSICALLY in comparison to the unrealistic expectations discussed? (Record these on a whiteboard.)

Examples

- *Possibly more muscular, or less if they are new to the sport*
- *Likely a higher (and healthier) body fat percentage*
- *Different heights (not as tall or short as the ideal)*
- *Smaller or larger breasts*
- *No one prototype—everyone is different ***Perhaps the most important take-home point*

How does an athlete with a healthy mindset and body image look MENTALLY and EMOTIONALLY in comparison to the unrealistic expectations discussed?

- *Views food as fuel for training and performance*
- *Is not scared of eating food and healthy weight gain*
- *Feels okay treating themselves to "unhealthy" foods that they enjoy*
- *Has a positive image of muscle tone and is proud to be strong OR of not having as much muscle volume as others—body confidence*
- *Has a positive image of her body in attaining goals (for swimming, running, basketball, general physical activity, etc.)*
- *Goals and nutrition are related to performance, improvement, and health rather than to the appearance of one's body*
- *Flexibility of mind to know that her body is not an indicator of who she is on the inside or of self-value*
- *Views athletes as all different sizes and shapes—knowing that ALL body types can excel in their sport*
- *Positive self-esteem*

What actions can athletes take to achieve their goals of aiming to have a healthy mindset and body image? Include psychological, emotional, and mental factors.

Examples

- *Steady attendance at practice*
- *Take pride in hard sets/workouts—even when they are tough*
- *Embrace all athletes as part of the team regardless of body type or other factors*
- *Eat nutrient-rich foods and make sure you are getting enough calories*
- *Prevent and take care of injuries (including not training through injuries)*
- *Lift weights and do strength work as appropriate*
- *Get adequate sleep*
- *Encourage teammates to view other female bodies in a positive manner*
- *Promote a culture accepting of every body type*
- *Recognize the difference between training hard and overexercising*

Who are some positive role model athletes who have a healthy attitude and prioritize their health and well-being over society's unrealistic ideals? What can we learn from them?

Varied answers

- *Simone Biles valued mental health at the Tokyo Olympics*
- *Serena Williams speaking out against stereotypical body types*
- *Norwegian beach handball wearing shorts instead of bikinis and being fined, but desiring practicality and modesty*
- *Paralympian runner Olivia Breen being ridiculed for wearing buns (tight short running shorts) and told it is too revealing, but competing in them as she feels more comfortable*
- *Germany's gymnastics team chose unitards at the Tokyo Olympics as they felt more comfortable*
- *Naomi Osaka, Japanese tennis star who pulled out of the French Open due to mental health*

NUTRITION (15 MINUTES)

Transition: Now, we will discuss how to use food to fuel your body for improved athletic performance and general well-being.

Discussion Questions (Leaders, please write answers on whiteboards/notepads.)

Why should we care about nutrition?

- *Nutrition as fuel for performance—performance in sports, classes, and life in general*
- *Provides energy for sports performance, health, and life*
- *Allows us to build muscle*

- *Allows us to recover after meets/games/hard practices*
- *Eating right can prevent certain health issues (cardiovascular disease, type II diabetes)*
- *Carries social and cultural value—enjoying holiday meals with family or post-competition milkshakes with the team is important, too*

What should we fuel with as female athletes?

- *Carbohydrates (pasta, bread, rice, quinoa, granola, etc.—aim for whole wheat or multigrain if possible)*
- *Fats (avocado, olive oil, coconut oil, etc.)*
- *Proteins (beef, chicken, pork, tofu, beans, fish, etc.)*
- *Veggies/Fruits (celery, broccoli, asparagus, apples, mangos, etc.)*
- *Vitamin/Minerals if we are not meeting certain needs in our diet (in particular calcium, vitamin D, and iron as female athletes)*
  - *Calcium and vitamin D = crucial in building strong bones and preventing bone injuries in addition to premature osteoporosis*
  - *Iron is necessary for helping our blood carry oxygen—low iron can be a common cause of fatigue in athletes, especially female athletes who lose iron during their menstrual cycle*

Why is breakfast important?

Leaders: Discuss cortisol response when female athletes do not eat breakfast—cortisol is a hormone produced by our bodies when under stress.

- *Our baseline cortisol is highest in the mornings. When we eat breakfast the cortisol levels go down. Skipping breakfast makes our bodies think we are in stress mode. When our body is in this perceived stress mode, we have a harder time regulating sugar levels, balancing our metabolism, and fighting infections*
- *By eating protein and carbs at breakfast, athletes can provide energy for afternoon practices*
- *Without breakfast, we can become tired by the afternoon, impacting our practices and performances*

What barriers may prevent someone from eating breakfast and how can we overcome these barriers?

- *Not enough time → Eat on the go (peanut butter toast with banana slices), prepare breakfast the night before (overnight oats)*
- *Not hungry → Start small and work your way up, try breakfast smoothies that contain all major food groups, and ask yourself if you are eating a large late-night snack that prevents you from eating breakfast the next morning*
- *Afraid of gaining weight → Gaining healthy weight is not a problem; it can also be muscle weight. Again, the cortisol response can be discussed.*

Healthy foods are the key to fueling well for our season, but they can be taken to the extreme. If we restrict our eating we can cause our bodies to be deprived of energy needed to improve performance. How can you balance eating healthy with also ensuring you are not restricting your nutrition or depriving yourself of your favorite foods?

- *Make sure to enjoy one treat a day (eating a piece of chocolate each night; having my favorite treat alongside a healthy meal)*
- *Having a milkshake with a healthy meal after a race; eating a healthy recovery snack, and having a treat*
- *Knowing it is okay to not have perfect nutrition and that it is a goal to work toward balanced and sustainable nutrition (sometimes you will have to be flexible with what you are eating and that is okay!)*
- *Recognizing that food has cultural and social context as well—enjoying holiday meals, ice cream with friends, or post-competition shakes with teammates is also part of healthy eating; eating should be balanced*

What should I eat before practice? And when should I try to eat before practice?

- *Carbohydrates and a little protein*
- *Snacks (banana or apple slices with peanut butter, protein balls, apple-sauce, dried fruit, trail mix, granola bar). If less than 45 minutes prior to practice, eat something more liquid with carbohydrates. If more than 60–90 minutes before practice, eat something with low fiber, low fat, and that is easy to digest. Granola, protein balls, or high-fat nut butter are less helpful this close to practice time. They are more appropriate 2–4 hours out especially for prone sports (swimming)*
- *Breakfast (bagel with peanut butter, oatmeal with fruit and peanut butter, peanut butter toast, Greek yogurt with an English muffin)*
- *Lunch (ham sandwich with apple slices, turkey wrap with veggies, chicken, and rice with cooked veggies)*
- *Dinner (chicken and rice burrito with salsa, spaghetti with meatballs, soup with a dinner roll)*

What should I eat to recover after practice?

- *Carbohydrates and protein as well as fluids*
- *Carbohydrates → Replenish energy stores depleted during exercise to quicken recovery and make sure you have sufficient energy for your next workout/competition*
- *Protein → Provides building blocks for muscle repair/growth*
- *Fluids → Replenish fluids lost in sweat during exercise*
- *Breakfast (eggs and toast/bagel, Greek yogurt and granola, pancakes with peanut butter or protein mix)*
- *Lunch/dinner (protein—chicken, pork, beef, tofu, beans; carbohydrates—rice, quinoa, bread, pasta)*

- *Snack (protein shake, chocolate milk, fruit with peanut butter or cheese sticks, celery, and peanut butter)*
- *Fluids (water, Gatorade, Nuun hydration tablets)—Can discuss tonicity of fluids if time. Electrolyte replacement? How long of exercise and how intense to need replacement? Under 1 hour this is likely not needed as water is enough.*

What should I eat prior to competition?

- *Focus on easily digested carbohydrates to provide quick energy for performance*
- *Ideally, use a snack/meal option you have tested out in practice*
- *Breakfast (bagel with apple slices, peanut butter toast with banana slices, oatmeal with berries)*
- *Lunch (turkey wrap, rice with lean chicken, lean beef, and rice burrito)*
- *Dinner (chicken noodle soup with dinner roll, spaghetti with meat sauce)*
- *Snacks (crackers, granola bar, trail mix, dried fruit, granola)*

RELATIVE ENERGY DEFICIENCY IN SPORT (10 MINUTES)

Leaders—Transition: To continue our discussion of nutrition, we want to talk about why it is so important that you, as athletes, ensure you are eating enough healthy calories to fuel yourselves for sport.

Discussion Questions

What do you feel like when you haven't eaten for a long time—when you feel "hangry"?

- *Irritable/crabby*
- *Tired/sleepy*
- *Weak/lacking energy*

What do you think would happen if you didn't eat enough over several days?

- *Tired/sleepy*
- *Weak/lacking energy*
- *Difficulty focusing in school or practice*
- *Difficulty remembering information*
- *The body breaks down muscle and bone for energy*

Do female athletes typically get enough calories?

Female athletes frequently underfuel in comparison to their athletic needs. Underfueling can lead to long-term issues in both athletics and your general health. This condition of underfueling is known as Relative Energy Deficiency in Sport (RED-S). We are going to go over a handout discussing the symptoms of RED-S and how we can avoid the development of RED-S.

RED-S Handout—Discussion Points

- *RED-S is multifactorial*
- *RED-S can lead to different outcomes in each athlete*
- *The severity of RED-S can vary widely*
- *Many aspects of RED-S can be reversed if dealt with early on*
- *Lifelong issues from RED-S can include fertility problems, poor bone density, and mental health issues (e.g. eating disorders, anxiety, depression)*
- *Bone density issues can be seen in teenagers (e.g. stress fractures and premature osteoporosis)*

HOMEWORK (5 MINUTES) * OPTIONAL—MAY OMIT IF TIME PROHIBITS

Homework: Come up with one nutrition goal and one mindset goal for positive change to work on. Write down five positive things about your body and mindset that help your performance.

Optional handouts

- Training Plate Activity
- Breakfast Importance
- Nutrition Myths vs. Facts

CONCLUSION (10 MINUTES)

Either end by doing a positive comments activity (athletes can randomly compliment teammates):

> *Does anyone want to say one last thing or compliment a teammate on a positive attribute they have seen in them?*

OR if time and athletes know each other, try a positivity circle:

> *One athlete sits in the middle and those surrounding say positive comments ranging from a time period of 30 seconds to 1 minute (depending on time restraints and group size). Have athletes take turns and ensure each person gets a chance to go who desires to participate.*

12 Handouts

Kathryn Vidlock

Rocky Vista University, Chambers Way, Parker, CO, USA

Catherine Liggett

University of Colorado School of Medicine, Aurora, CO, USA

CONTENTS

THE TRAINING PLATE MODEL

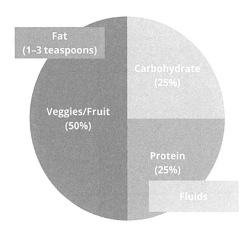

DOI: 10.1201/b23228-12

Low-Intensity Training Plate

Intended for rest days or light recovery days (e.g. stretching, walking, yoga).

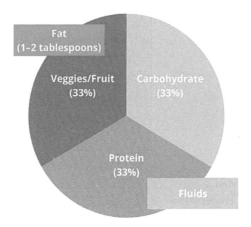

Moderate-Intensity Training Plate

Intended for "baseline" training (e.g. skills-based practice with lifting afterwards or a base run/swim).

High-Intensity Training Plate

Intended for strenuous workouts (e.g. long run or high-intensity interval work, two-a-day and pre-competition/competition fueling).

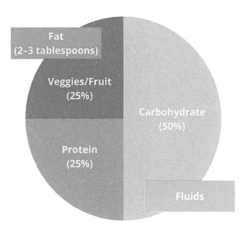

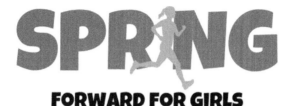

FORWARD FOR GIRLS

Strength and Positivity
Rooted in Nutrition for Girls

HOMEWORK SESSION 1

IG: @spring_forward_girls

Homework: Come up with one nutrition goal and one mindset goal for positive change to work on in between this session and our next. Write down five positive things about your body and mindset that help your performance.

Nutrition Goal:

Mindset Goal:

Five positive things about my body and mindset. (Make sure you have at least one for body and one for mindset.)

1.

2.

3.

4.

5.

RELATIVE ENERGY DEFICIENCY IN SPORT (RED-S)

Playing a sport requires a significant amount of energy from your body. Just think about how tired your body feels after a hard workout, lifting session, or competition. How do you think your body would feel if you had to do those activities after skipping meals all day? What if you had skipped multiple meals for the past week?

If your answer to the above questions was "probably not so good", you are spot on! Athletes who practice or compete with low energy are not able to perform to their best ability. Not only does athletic performance suffer but your health can too. Athletes who underfuel their bodies for sport (aka athletes who are burning more energy than they are consuming) are prone to suffer from a condition called **Relative Energy Deficiency in Sport (RED-S)**.

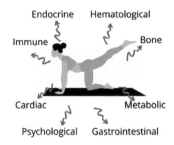

If an athlete burns more energy than they consume, their body will enter a **low-energy state**. In RED-S, an individual experiences low energy levels due to improper fueling for sport. Our body is able to recognize this low-energy state and responds by attempting to conserve energy. Our body does this by dysregulating "less important" organ systems (e.g. the reproductive system) to conserve energy for "more important" organ systems (e.g. the brain or heart).

For female athletes, the first sign of RED-S is often missed or irregular periods. This is because the reproductive system is generally one of the first organ systems to be dysregulated in a low-energy state. At first glance, this may sound like great news—who wants an annoying and uncomfortable period each month anyways?

The problem with this is that periods are actually incredibly important to female health. When we have our period each month, our body also releases an important hormone called **estrogen**. In biological females, estrogen is crucial to building strong bones. For athletes who miss their period, estrogen is no longer released. Over time, this leads to weakening of the bones and increased risk of **bone injuries** (e.g. fractures, stress fractures, premature osteoporosis).

90% of bone mass is achieved by age 18 in biological females. If you have weak bones at age 18 due to underfueling for sport, you are increasing your risk of lifelong bone health issues.

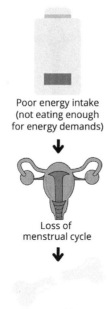

Poor energy intake
(not eating enough
for energy demands)

Loss of
menstrual cycle

Decreased bone
density & increased
risk of bone injury

If an athlete stays in a low-energy state for an extended period of time, they may begin to experience body-wide performance and health issues as more organ systems become dysregulated to save energy. Some of these performance and health conditions can be reversed with proper fueling, while others can have more permanent impacts. This combination of performance and health issues due to low energy is RED-S.

Factors increasing risk of RED-S include but are not limited to:

- **Being an athlete**: Athletes have higher energy demands than their nonathletic peers because of the additional energy needed to fuel sport.
- **Athletes in middle school and high school**: It takes energy to grow! Youth athletes have higher energy requirements to support growth and development (puberty).
- **Athletes in certain sports**: Sports that foster false perceptions of weight loss as necessary for sport performance, beliefs of how an athlete should look for their sport, or weight classification requirements to compete are at an elevated risk of RED-S (e.g. endurance sports, gymnastics, figure skating, dance, wrestling).

After hearing all this, you are probably wondering how you can prevent and/or treat RED-S. **Prevention and treatment of RED-S means addressing the root issue— low energy levels**.

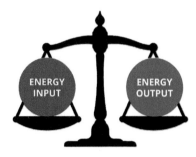

When thinking of energy deficiency in athletes there are two factors to consider: energy input and energy output. Energy input can be increased by eating enough to fuel energy demands and engaging in more consistent fueling habits. If nutrition habits are not enough to address energy deficiency (e.g. you are working on improved nutrition but still not having your period), energy output can be decreased by reducing physical activity and/or prioritizing rest. RED-S is due to an energy imbalance, and in order to appropriately prevent/treat RED-S, this energy imbalance must be addressed directly through nutrition and exercise habits.

It is important to note that athletes with missing periods due to RED-S may be recommended to use birth control in order to regulate their menstrual cycles. This is NOT an appropriate way to treat RED-S. Birth control produces a synthetic period without addressing underlying energy imbalance issues. In effect, birth control causes an athlete to have a "pill-induced" period but does not address the actual underlying energy imbalance issues. This may lead an athlete to believe their problem with RED-S is solved when it really is not. Because energy imbalance is not addressed with birth control, the athlete may still experience the negative performance and health issues associated with RED-S. With this being said, there are many other reasons to be on birth control—always have a conversation with your healthcare provider before starting or ceasing any treatment plan.

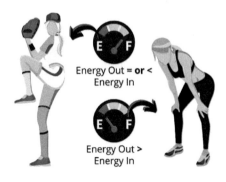

Energy Out = **or** <
Energy In

Energy Out >
Energy In

Overall, RED-S is prevented and treated by addressing energy deficit issues. RED-S is a serious condition that can have numerous performance and health impacts that in certain cases can be long term. If you are struggling with RED-S, reach out to a healthcare provider who is knowledgeable about treatment of RED-S in order to get connected with the appropriate resources.

"EATING WELL IS A FORM OF SELF-RESPECT"

IG: @spring_forward_girls

Nutrition Basics

Let's strive for a mindset of food as fuel for your performance in practice and competition. What do we need? Macronutrients (carbohydrates, proteins, and fats) are essential.

Carbohydrates are natural sugars and starches in grain foods (breads, cereal, pasta) and vegetables, fruits, beans, and legumes. The sugar in candy, sweets, and some sport drinks are simple carbohydrates and lack the nutrient value of more complex carbohydrates. Our bodies store extra carbohydrates as glycogen. We use these stores during workouts, so a deficiency in glycogen stores will make us tired and performance will suffer. **Proteins** are made of amino acids and help with building muscles. Sources of protein include meats, fish, eggs, beans, and nuts. **Fats** are necessary, but eating fats with nutrients will increase performance. Good sources include nuts, avocados, and some dairy items.

How do we use these sources in various scenarios?

Breakfast: Breakfast is especially important for female athletes. A breakfast containing protein will help you feel strong at afternoon practices. Include some complex carbohydrates to keep your glycogen stores strong. Good examples include toast with eggs, cereal with milk, oatmeal with yogurt and fruit, and granola with fruit.

Fast fuel before practice after school or before competition: Some carbohydrates that are easily digested are best for this timing. Examples include a piece of fruit, granola bar, or crackers. Eating a snack high in simple carbohydrates might give you a quick burst of energy but will drop your sugar level shortly and you may feel tired at practice.

Quick recovery fuel after practice if you aren't going to have a meal soon: If the timing means a quick snack instead of mealtime, here are some options: string cheese, crackers and fruit; pretzels and chocolate milk.

After a hard practice: For recovery a female athlete needs both carbohydrates and proteins to replenish glycogen stores and build muscle. Many experts say a 3:1 ratio of carbohydrates for recovery is best. Examples include pasta with meatballs and sauce and a vegetable, French toast with eggs, deli sandwich with a side of fruit, or baked potato with chicken and a vegetable. Chocolate milk is a popular and nutritious recovery drink option.

Pre-competition meal—The night before: The night before a competition is not a good time to try something new and spicy. Eat something with carbohydrates and some protein. Examples include pasta with red sauce or rice with poultry and vegetables. If you have trouble with your stomach during competition, avoid too much fiber the day before and day of the event. Drink plenty of fluids the day before.

Pre-competition—The day of the event: If the event is in the morning, good choices include easy-to-digest carbohydrates like a bagel or cereal or a fruit smoothie. If the event is later in the day, add more protein to breakfast and then have either a quick snack before a mid-day competition or a lunch rich in carbohydrates for an event later in the day. Keep drinking fluids during the day.

Prior to your big event—Carb loading: Endurance athletes tapering for a big season-end event should consider carb loading. While tapering, athletes may need to cut back a little on eating as they are exercising less. Starting two days before the event, eat foods rich in carbohydrates. Drinking plenty of fluids is also necessary. Again, you will want to have some protein and fat, but concentrate on carbohydrates as the main portion. Examples include French toast and fruit, bagel and peanut butter, rice and vegetables, macaroni salad, sandwiches and fruit, vegetable soups, pasta and sauce, popcorn, and crackers.

What about letting myself splurge? It is fine to let yourself have the things you love. Considering the timing will allow you to have these yummy treats and still fuel properly for the season. If you want a cupcake, wait until after the competition and make sure you also have some appropriate fuel for recovery. Craving some fast food? Maybe an off day is the best option.

THE IMPORTANCE OF BREAKFAST FOR ATHLETES

So you know getting in each meal as an athlete is important. But what makes breakfast in particular so important for athletes? Let's get into the science behind it!

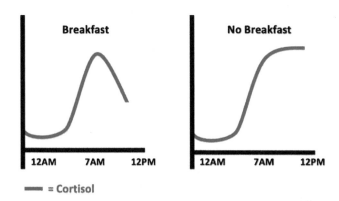

Cortisol levels peak in the early morning. Eating breakfast causes these levels to drop, but if you skip breakfast, these levels are maintained which is associated with negative health outcomes.

It all starts with a hormone called **cortisol**. Cortisol is released from our body in times of **stress**. When we think of stress, we may draw negative associations; however, stress (to a certain degree) is actually important and beneficial to our health. Our body may experience stress when we push ourselves in a hard workout or when we've gone too long without eating.

These "stress" situations are not necessarily dangerous as long as we don't push our body too far past its limitations. In this way, think of stress as a sign or signal to our body.

As we sleep overnight, our body enters a **fasted state**—a period of time without eating. As the night progresses, this "stress" of not eating elevates. As stress increases, levels of cortisol (that "stress" hormone we talked about earlier) also increase. By the time your body is ready to awaken in the morning, you have reached a pretty noticeable elevation in cortisol levels. This elevation in cortisol levels is actually what induces your body to wake rather than continue to sleep. Biological females tend to have higher baseline cortisol levels in the morning than biological males. It is important to note this phenomenon is more widely researched in adult populations.

This increase in cortisol levels sounds like a good thing—and it is when it comes to waking us up in the morning! After eating breakfast, cortisol levels decrease because the stress of not eating for an extended period of time has now been removed. Removal of the "stressor" leads to a reduction in cortisol levels. Now ask yourself—what would happen to these cortisol levels if you skipped breakfast?

Breakfast Tips & Tricks

1. Try an option you can prepare the night before to save time in the morning (e.g. overnight oats).

2. It doesn't have to be fancy—go for a simple and quick breakfast option in the morning (e.g. peanut butter toast topped with banana slices.

3. Start small—if you are getting used to eating breakfast in the morning for the first time, try something small (e.g. a piece of fruit).

4. Utilize liquid options like smoothies or breakfast shakes if you struggle with an appetite in the morning.

That's right! If you don't eat breakfast in the morning after waking up, then cortisol levels do not go down until your first meal of the day—which for many busy athletes (who tend to be rushed in the morning) may not be until lunch. This presents a problem for us. Elevated cortisol levels for an extended period of time have negative implications for both athletic performance and health. For this reason, getting breakfast when you wake up in the morning is crucial to regulation of cortisol levels.

For those who find themselves too rushed in the morning to eat, try quick breakfast options like overnight oats or peanut butter toast with banana slices on top. If you struggle with an appetite in the morning, train your gut by starting small—something is better than nothing. Alternatively, utilize liquid options like smoothies or breakfast shakes. We know getting breakfast in can be difficult, but it is well worth the time to improve your athletic performance and health.

HOMEWORK SESSION 2

IG: @spring_forward_girls

Find a private spot and read aloud the positive things you wrote about yourself from last time. If you did not write anything down from last time, write your five positive items first.

Was it difficult to read the positive things aloud? Was this harder than just writing them down?

Write a new nutrition goal and positive body image goal as well as a sleep goal.

New Nutrition Goal:

New Mindset Goal:

Sleep Goal:

NUTRITION MYTHS

IG: @spring_forward_girls

The Myth	The Fact
Eating carbohydrates will make you gain weight.	Carbohydrates are necessary to replenish energy stores to fuel performance.
Vegetarian diets are healthier than nonvegetarian diets.	Both vegetarian and nonvegetarian diets can be either healthy or nonhealthy depending on the choices.
During the season, you should never eat unhealthy foods.	It is okay to treat yourself with the unhealthy foods you like—just try to time these after practice and meets.
You should avoid fat in your diet to stay skinny.	You need some fat in your diet to stay healthy. You should get 20–35% of calories from fat sources.

(Continued)

The Myth	The Fact
Gatorade and Powerade are always healthy fueling choices.	If you are working out over an hour, replacing electrolytes is recommended. Both Powerade and Gatorade contain sugar, which may be needed in some cases of exercise, but drinking these types of drinks throughout the day is unnecessary.
I should never eat the unhealthy treats I love.	Having a diet that is too strict is not healthy for your body or mind. You can have the things you enjoy.
There is one magic diet that works for every single athlete.	Each athlete should work to improve their diet on an individual basis. Everybody has different needs.
Vitamin supplements give you "quick" energy.	While some vitamins and minerals can help with metabolism, they are not forms of "quick" energy.

13 Parent Information

Kathryn Vidlock

Rocky Vista University, Chambers Way, Parker, CO, USA

Catherine Liggett

University of Colorado School of Medicine, Aurora, CO, USA

CONTENTS

WHAT IF MY CHILD SEEMS IN IMMINENT DANGER?

This book is in no way a substitute for professional help. If your child is in imminent danger either call 9-1-1 or 9-8-8, if your area has mental health services, or go to the nearest emergency department.

If your child is in imminent danger, either call **9-1-1 or 9-8-8** if your areas has mental health services, or go to the nearest emergency department.

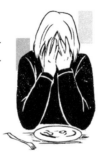

DOI: 10.1201/b23228-13

If you are a parent reading this and have made it this far into the book, then you are already working towards being a parent promoting the well-being of your child.

HOW BIG IS THE PROBLEM?

According to the National Association of Anorexia Nervosa and Associated Disorders (ANAD), the statistics show this is a huge problem. Eating disorders affect 9% of the US population. Twenty-six percent of those with an eating disorder will attempt suicide.[1] In our experience working with teens, almost every teen either has some risk factors or has a close friend who has experienced risk factors. Risk factors alone do not mean they will go on to have a diagnosed eating disorder, and parents can play a role in encouraging healthy eating and body image habits.

BUT MY CHILD SEEMS AN APPROPRIATE WEIGHT

Unfortunately, weight is not an indicator. Of those diagnosed with an eating disorder, less than 6% are underweight.[2] Many athletes with normal weights have binge eating disorder or bulimia risk factors or symptoms.

WHAT IF MY CHILD SUDDENLY WANTS TO EAT HEALTHIER?

This might be a normal healthy reaction to being an athlete and desiring a healthy body. Healthy eating in and of itself is fine. But if taken to the extreme, it can be unhealthy. Orthorexia is a term for when healthy eating becomes so extreme that it is unhealthy. Watch for an athlete that is skipping meals or wants to always eat alone. Encourage them to eat a variety of foods.

WHAT IS THE RIGHT AMOUNT OF EXERCISING?

One of the red flags to watch for is athletes that exercise outside of their practice time. But, sometimes athletes will need to do extra work including weight lifting or practice on their own as directed by their coach. The red flag is when an athlete is doing more than what their coach recommends. Another warning sign is when an athlete uses food as a reward only when a certain level of exercise is done. Athletes should fuel properly even on rest days. One caveat is that if they have a particularly hard workout then they may need more food or fuel. Keep in mind that their mindset is key. Looking at food as extra fuel for a hard workout is different than only allowing oneself to have an extra cookie or snack if they burn so many calories. Exercising through injuries is another red flag. If they continue to run on a stress fracture, clearly there is a problem. However, moving to an exercise such as swimming or biking or something deemed safe to do in the midst of the specific injury is a healthy approach.

STRESS

Teens' lives are more stressful than in years past. The stresses in school, work, teams and friend relationships seem overwhelming at times. Mental illnesses are alarmingly high in teenagers. Stress can contribute to a teen's likelihood to experience eating disorder symptoms. Parents should watch their children especially in times of stress.

Normalize talking about mental health issues in your family. Mental health issues in teenagers have risen drastically in the past ten years. It may be in part because we are better at recognizing symptoms. Even with the increased recognition and media attention, there is a stigma associated with having depression, anxiety, or an eating disorder. There is a lot of guilt and shame associated with any mental illness. But it is just that—an illness. We would treat other chronic diseases with care and support. As parents, talk about mental health issues with your children. Almost every family has a member who deals with some sort of mental issue. The more we discuss and normalize things, the better the treatment will become.

HOW DO I TALK TO MY TEEN ABOUT THIS?

One thing that teenagers want, almost universally, is respect. They respond best to respectful conversations.

Make a plan before you start talking; write down talking points if desired. Approaching them with statistics may just lead to eye rolling. Directly asking them if they have an eating disorder may just lead to denial, although sometimes asking the question can be a way to open the conversation, if the child and parent have a relationship where that feels supportive. Talking openly and sharing your concerns is often the best approach. Explain that adults may not have endured the same types of stress that this generation feels, but the adults are no strangers to stress. Be empathetic above all. Talk to them about the dangers of dieting instead of specific disordered eating behaviors. Ask them questions and don't lecture. Encourage positive habits and point out some things they do that are positive. Above all, promote flexible thinking.

Parents modeling flexibility and healthy habits is very important. Don't complain that you don't look good in your swimsuit. Don't label foods as only good and bad. Teach balanced eating as well as a flexible approach to foods. Foods we consider bad may have some nutritional value and a place as a fun food or a traditional holiday food.

Accept all body types and talk about healthy and athletic bodies coming in all shapes and sizes. There are many incredibly skilled athletes who look bigger than nonathletic people. These bigger bodies are likely healthier, yet get a bad rap because society associates thinness with beauty. Talk openly about society's influence on body image disorders. Large corporations prey on body image disorders by photoshopping already-thin models. Make sure your child sees the hypocritical money-making desires behind these ads.

It is generally better to have deep discussions while there is no food involved. Make sure both parties are calm and receptive to interacting. If not, choose another time. These conversations can be very emotional, so remember to stay calm and respectful and take a break if needed.

Above all, do not comment on their body. If they have concerns, keep your comments about body diversity. Explain that we all have different bodies and that no one body type is superior or inferior. Ask them what they like about their body, how does it perform, what features does their body provide that help them athletically? Strong heart? Muscular legs for speed?

WHAT IF MY CHILD IS NOT ON A TEAM OR THEIR SCHOOL DOESN'T USE THIS PROGRAM?

You can certainly read through the manuals with your child. Even better, if they have someone closer to their age who is a role model, that might be a good option to go over this information with them. If possible, include some friends or teammates so that the discussion doesn't all fall to one athlete.

WHAT IF I HAVE WITNESSED SOME RED FLAG SYMPTOMS?

Be very careful with the discussion here. Starting with accusatory statements usually does not go well. Asking calm questions leading up to the behaviors is usually more productive. Don't act embarrassed or shame your child. Make sure they feel comfortable and that you are there to listen. Explain that eating disorders are a real disease and that they can ask for help. Remember that there are a lot of self-esteem issues tied to eating disorders.

If your child has an eating disorder, get help. Involve your child in the plan for help. They are much more likely to follow a plan that they helped choose. This is very unlikely to get better without professional help. You can start with a physician or mental health provider, but will likely have to get both involved. Treatment of an eating disorder is best done with a multifactorial plan including the athlete, parents, coaches, physician, and psychologist and/or psychiatrist.

Don't use anger or try to scare them out of their behaviors. Don't force them to eat with the family. This approach will likely backfire. It is wiser to show you care and open the door to conversations.

You may not have to stop their athletic activities. This depends on the severity of the eating disorder. Getting help from professionals is the first step and they can help you decide if a break from athletics is the best option or not.

AN ATHLETE'S STORY: Krista

I joined the volleyball team in middle school. I wasn't very good but I made friends with the team's star, Emily. We became best friends very quickly. She loved volleyball and gave me tips and we both made JV our freshman year. Emily loved to eat and she never gained weight. I noticed I was putting on weight with all the junk food we ate together. I asked Emily what she was doing. I thought maybe she was running or something. But she wasn't. She made me promise not to tell anyone. She was making herself throw up after eating. Over the next several months she showed me websites where girls shared secrets on how to stay thin. We used laxatives, diuretics, and binged and purged. I thought it was great. We could eat whatever we wanted.

Emily started restricting her diet because she felt fat. She didn't seem any different to me. I restricted my diet. We learned how to suck on ice cubes instead of eating and filled up with tons of water. It worked and we lost weight.

Our volleyball uniforms looked so good on us. Our classmates said we looked like models. Emily stopped getting her period, and I desperately wanted that. A few months later, it stopped.

We lied to parents, friends, coaches, our doctors, and anyone else who asked about our eating. Our parents were still worried. Parents have no idea how much information is available on the internet. We found other girls doing the same things. We shared ways to hide it from our family and friends. Our volleyball skills were getting worse and we were tired. But we didn't care, we looked great—or so we thought.

Then my world came crashing down. I was about to leave for school one morning when we received a call. Emily had been found dead in her bed that morning by her parents. My best friend was gone. It wasn't suicide. There was no note. Her doctors believed it was a heart problem brought on by anorexia.

I was inconsolable. I felt in a fog for weeks. I couldn't think. I just walked through the motions of my day. She was gone. Never coming back. Worse yet— it could have just as easily been me. What was I doing?

I came clean about everything to my parents. I told Emily's parents everything. They blamed themselves for not forcing her to get help. It would not have mattered—we were getting too many compliments from our peers. My parents wanted me to have inpatient help for the eating disorder and see a psychologist to help with the loss of Emily. I agreed. I took a semester off from high school. My counselors and teachers were very supportive.

It has been 12 years since her death. I think of her often, especially when eating some of our favorite foods. Her death was completely preventable. Sometimes I am sad about it and other times I am angry. What is wrong with our society that we place emphasis on model-like figures? What does it take to change that value? Why do we continue to value a skinny little teen body? We, as a society, are literally killing our own children. We support big corporations that perpetuate this image of stick thin models with large breasts and a Barbie-like figure that isn't realistic. It has to stop. Girls, we need to support each other.

This project is so important. I don't know if this project would have changed our attitudes or prevented Emily's death. But I hope every girl participating finds the confidence to stand up to archaic societal values and remain positive about themselves.

CITATIONS

1. Arcelus J, Mitchell AJ, Wales J, Nielsen S. Mortality Rates in Patients with Anorexia Nervosa and Other Eating Disorders. A Meta-Analysis of 36 Studies. *Arch Gen Psychiatry.* 2011; 68(7): 724–731.
2. Flament MF, Henderson K, Buchholz A et al. Weight Status and DSM-5 Diagnoses of Eating Disorders in Adolescents from the Community. *J Am Acad Child Adolesc Psychiatry.* 2015; 54(5): 403–411.e2. doi:10.1016/j.jaac.2015.01.020

14 Social Media

Catherine Liggett

University of Colorado School of Medicine, Aurora, CO, USA

Kathryn Vidlock

Rocky Vista University, Parker, CO, USA

CONTENTS

High school is a time in which young girls transition from adolescence to adulthood and subsequently develop their own personal perceptions regarding a healthy and balanced approach to eating, exercise, and body image. The beliefs established during this time can be sustained throughout adulthood, making high school an opportune period to ensure young girls are engaging in behaviors that promote long-term, sustainable health benefits.

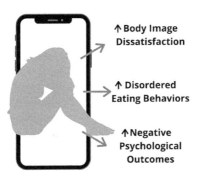

↑ Body Image Dissatisfaction

↑ Disordered Eating Behaviors

↑ Negative Psychological Outcomes

SOCIAL MEDIA ROLE IN BODY IMAGE

Over the past decades, social media has become a predominant platform in which high school girls can establish an online identity and then gather information, refine individual viewpoints, and interact with others. While the expansion of social media platforms has allowed for increased dissemination of educational tools and access to a variety of global resources, social media has also been shown to precipitate increased rates of body image dissatisfaction, heightened risk of disordered eating behaviors, and other negative psychological outcomes.[1, 2]

Due to the largely unregulated nature of social media, nutrition and health professionals often find themselves fighting the proliferation of false beauty and nutrition perceptions as promoted by fitness "influencers", celebrity endorsements, or mass marketing campaigns from corporate food and health brands. "Fitspiration", which consists of images, quotes, and/or advice pertaining to exercise and eating may or may not promote the best health guidance for young female athletes, dependent upon the source. In one study, 17.7% of participants who regularly accessed "fitspiration" content were shown to be at high risk for an eating disorder while 17.4% reported high levels of psychological distress.[3] Accessibility and ease of use with Photoshop editing apps has also created misconstrued ideologies of beauty that can be difficult to discern from more realistic body standards for young girls. The issue has even gone so far as to push a proposal of legislation that would require a disclaimer under images utilizing Photoshop.

The 2021 Pew Research Center survey on social media use showed 95% of young adults utilize some form of social media with the highest rates of use being attributed to Instagram (76%) and TikTok (55%).[4] Visual-based social media platforms, such as Instagram, have been attributed to greater body dissatisfaction and weight loss behaviors. Exposure to edited images of celebrities and/or peers alongside "fitspiration" posts often praise thinness and extreme fitness levels which, when internalized, have been linked with poor body image perceptions.[5]

USING SOCIAL MEDIA IN A POSITIVE WAY

Due to the high use of Instagram among young women in addition to the body image risks associated with visual-based social media platforms, we chose to utilize Instagram for social media outreach with SPRING Forward for Girls (@spring_forward_girls). Our hope in creating a social media page was to directly communicate with high school athletes, while also providing more balanced eating, exercise, and body image content on the Instagram feed of our followers.

To combat internalized perceptions of unsustainable body ideals as acquired from social media, we recommend athletes be selective when deciding which pages to follow. Particularly, we advise athletes to unfollow pages promoting unrealistic body ideals and disordered eating/exercise behaviors, replacing these pages with ones such as SPRING Forward for Girls in addition to other body-positive social media accounts. By following pages committed to balanced and sustainable lifestyle approaches, athletes can better garner the positive effects of social media use while avoiding negative outcomes.

For high school teams, clubs, or other groups utilizing the SPRING Forward for Girls program, we recommend creation of a social media page specific to your association and then linking this with our organization's page. It can be helpful to assign the social media page to the team. Pick a SPRING Forward Ambassador or someone who is interested in social media and is a positive role model. By doing this, each group utilizing the program should have access to their own social media page with specific program updates, reminders, etc., while also being able to access the resources and information provided from our social media page. The athlete can repost from the SPRING social media or similar places and provide specific tips for various times of the season or make the nutrition information correlate to the team's specific schedule. This approach should allow athletes to connect with fellow teammates via their local Instagram page in addition to interacting globally with the SPRING Forward for Girls community at large.

In addition, feel free to use a little of the session time to discuss something trending on social media. It can either be positive or negative. The important part is recognizing the impact that social media has. By recognizing it for its honesty or dishonesty, the athletes learn to apply the principles taught here.

PREVALENCE OF SOCIAL MEDIA USE AMONG HIGH SCHOOLERS

Many teenagers utilize social media of some form whether on platforms such as Instagram, Snapchat, Twitter, or TikTok. The Pew Research Center's most recent survey on teens and social media use shows the following:

BENEFITS OF SOCIAL MEDIA USE FOR ATHLETES

- Connecting with family and friends
- Navigating reputable information sources
- Meeting other individuals with similar interests
- A form of entertainment
- A way to self-express and share personal interests
- Finding support from other individuals
- Learning new things

RISKS OF SOCIAL MEDIA USE FOR ATHLETES

- Cyberbullying
- Difficulty communicating online rather than in person
- Harms certain relationships
- Provides unrealistic view on other users' lives
- Creates unrealistic perceptions on how an individual should eat, exercise, look, etc.
- Distracts or leads to constant usage of social media
- Contributes to peer pressure and "fitting in"
- Increases risk of certain mental health issues

In addition to the Instagram page, SPRING Forward has a Facebook page and website. We realize that teens are more likely to follow Instagram and other more visual social media. However, Facebook and the website do provide information that is useful for all, including coaches, adult athletes, parents, athletic trainers, and others involved.

We encourage adults to pay attention to what their teenage athletes are following on their social media. Ask them to share videos or positive posts with you. Clearly, this will not keep them from experiencing negative posts and videos, but it will highlight some of the positive messages that can come from social media. Encourage them to share negative posts with you also. You can discuss the negative message. Some teens will feel empowered by commenting on negative posts or videos. Each family needs to make their own decisions on social media usage, but in general, we discourage a total ban. Usually that results in teens just finding other means to see social media. It is usually better to allow it and monitor it as available.

AN ATHLETE'S STORY: Charlotte

My varsity running shorts were really short—so short that my butt cheeks showed. I didn't want to look fat. Some girls commented that I was the large girl on the team. That hurt me so deeply. I wanted to look like the elite runners with very skinny legs. They had no cheeks to show. My whole family is big boned, and I felt if I dieted enough, I could overcome it. I ate less and less. When I was hungry, I ate ice chips. I started avoiding dinners.

I became skinner and took pride in looking in the mirror and seeing the thin arms and legs. But I felt awful. No matter what I did, I could not lose my cheeks. I tried specific butt exercises but that just seems to make them stronger, not skinnier. My times got better at first, then they got worse. I started caring more about getting skinny legs than the times. I couldn't be both faster and skinny. People complimented my weight loss. I found sites on the internet where girls were power dieting and I did everything they did to get skinnier. I was so obsessed with eating. If I ate a cookie, I ran 5 miles to punish myself. I never achieved any fast times.

I spent most of my freshman year in college partying and not eating food at all. I felt sick but I thought I looked great. My feelings of decreased self-worth all went away when I drank. I spent most of that year not eating but drinking heavily and throwing up. I hit rock bottom when I got a DWI. I felt alone and sick and slowly realized that I wasn't who I wanted to be. Everyone was mad at me— my parents, my friends. I knew I needed to pull it together, but I wasn't sure how.

I joined a group for those with eating disorders. Slowly I learned how bad the damage was to myself. I started seeing a therapist. My parents were upset that I saw a therapist because they didn't want anyone to know I had a mental illness. Once I got my own insurance they didn't have to know anymore. I finished college and started running again, but I had learned to stay in a different frame of mind. Running became a form of relaxation and pleasure, not a way to beat up my body to burn more calories.

I still struggle but I am doing better. I don't want other girls to ever feel this way. I wish I had never listened to the insults of high school girls. My life could have been so much different if I had more confidence then.

CITATIONS

1. Yang, Hwajin et al. "Effects of Social Media and Smartphone Use on Body Esteem in Female Adolescents: Testing a Cognitive and Affective Model." *Children (Basel, Switzerland)*, 21 Sep. 2020; 7(9): 148. doi:10.3390/children7090148.
2. Jiotsa, Barbara et al. "Social Media Use and Body Image Disorders: Association between Frequency of Comparing One's Own Physical Appearance to That of People Being Followed on Social Media and Body Dissatisfaction and Drive for Thinness." *International Journal of Environmental Research and Public Health*, 11 Mar. 2021;18(6): 2880. doi:10.3390/ijerph18062880.
3. Raggatt, Michelle et al. "'I aspire to look and feel healthy like the posts convey': Engagement with Fitness Inspiration on Social Media and Perceptions of Its Influence on Health and Wellbeing." *BMC Public Health*, 10 Aug. 2018;18(1): 1002, doi:10.1186/s12889-018-5930-7.
4. Auxier, B. & Anderson, M. "Social Media Use in 2021: A Majority of Americans Say They Use YouTube and Facebook, While Use of Instagram, Snapchat and TikTok Is Especially Common among Adults under 30." *Pew Research Center*, April 7, 2021.
5. Rounsefell, Kim et al. "Social Media, Body Image and Food Choices in Healthy Young Adults: A Mixed Methods Systematic Review." *Nutrition & Dietetics: The Journal of the Dietitians Association of Australia*, 2020;77(1): 19–40. doi:10.1111/1747-0080.12581.

Index

Page numbers in *italics* indicate figures. Page numbers in **bold** indicate tables.